T0362430

Optimizing Endoscopic Operations

Editors

SUNGUK N. JANG
JOHN J. VARGO

GASTROINTESTINAL ENDOSCOPY CLINICS OF NORTH AMERICA

www.giendo.theclinics.com

Consulting Editor
CHARLES J. LIGHTDALE

October 2021 • Volume 31 • Number 4

ELSEVIER

1600 John F. Kennedy Boulevard • Suite 1800 • Philadelphia, Pennsylvania, 19103-2899

http://www.theclinics.com

GASTROINTESTINAL ENDOSCOPY CLINICS OF NORTH AMERICA Volume 31, Number 4
October 2021 ISSN 1052-5157, ISBN-13: 978-0-323-81357-0

Editor: Kerry Holland
Developmental Editor: Jessica Cañaberal

Gastrointestinal Endoscopy Clinics of North America (ISSN 1052-5157) is published quarterly by Elsevier Inc., 360 Park Avenue South, New York, NY 10010-1710. Months of issue are January, April, July, and October. Business and Editorial Offices: 1600 John F. Kennedy Blvd., Suite 1800, Philadelphia, PA, 19103-2899. Periodicals postage paid at New York, NY and additional mailing offices. Subscription prices are $363.00 per year for US individuals, $813.00 per year for US institutions, $100.00 per year for US and Canadian students/residents, $399.00 per year for Canadian individuals, $841.00 per year for Canadian institutions, $476.00 per year for international individuals, $841.00 per year for international institutions, and $245.00 per year for international students/residents. To receive student/resident rate, orders must be accompanied by name of affiliated institution, date of term, and the *signature* of program/residency coordinator on institution letterhead. Orders will be billed at individual rate until proof of status is received. Foreign air speed delivery is included in all *Clinics* subscription prices. All prices are subject to change without notice. **POSTMASTER:** Send address change to *Gastrointestinal Endoscopy Clinics of North America*, Elsevier Health Sciences Division, Subscription Customer Service, 3251 Riverport Lane, Maryland Heights, MO 63043. **Customer Service: 1-800-654-2452 (US). From outside the United States, call 1-314-447-8871. Fax: 1-314-447-8029. E-mail: JournalsCustomerService-usa@elsevier.com (for print support) or JournalsOnlineSupport-usa@elsevier.com (for online support).**

Reprints. For copies of 100 or more, of articles in this publication, please contact the Commercial Reprints Department, Elsevier Inc., 360 Park Avenue South, New York, NY 10010-1710. Tel. 212-633-3874; Fax: 212-633-3820; E-mail: reprints@elsevier.com.

Gastrointestinal Endoscopy Clinics of North America is covered in *Excerpta Medica, MEDLINE/PubMed (Index Medicus), and MEDLINE/MEDLARS.*

Contributors

CONSULTING EDITOR

CHARLES J. LIGHTDALE, MD
Professor of Medicine, Division of Digestive and Liver Diseases, Columbia University Medical Center, New York, New York

EDITORS

SUNGUK N. JANG, MD
Associate Director, Enterprise Endoscopy Operation, Associate Professor, Case Western Reserve University School of Medicine, Associate Section Head, Advanced Endoscopy, Department of Gastroenterology, Hepatology and Nutrition, Digestive Disease and Surgery Institute, Cleveland Clinic, Cleveland, Ohio, USA

JOHN J. VARGO, MD, MPH, MASGE, AGAF, FACP, FACG, FGJES
Director, Enterprise Endoscopy Operations, Director, Endoscopic Research and Innovation, Head, Section of Advanced Endoscopy, Department of Gastroenterology, Hepatology and Nutrition, Digestive Disease and Surgery Institute, Cleveland Clinic, Associate Professor of Medicine, Cleveland Clinic Lerner College of Medicine, Case Western Reserve University, Cleveland, Ohio, USA

AUTHORS

ASYIA AHMAD, MD, MPH
Professor of Medicine, Division of Gastroenterology, Drexel University College of Medicine/Tower Health Medical Group, Philadelphia, Pennsylvania, USA

TYLER M. BERZIN, MD, MS, FASGE
Center for Advanced Endoscopy, Division of Gastroenterology and Hepatology, Beth Israel Deaconess Medical Center, Harvard Medical School, Boston, Massachusetts, USA

KATHY BULL-HENRY, MD
Medical Director, Endoscopy Unit, Johns Hopkins Bayview Hospital, Johns Hopkins Medicine, Baltimore, Maryland, USA

AUSTIN L. CHIANG, MD, MPH
Assistant Professor of Medicine, Sidney Kimmel Medical College, Director, Endoscopic Bariatric Program, Thomas Jefferson University Hospital, Chief Medical Social Media Officer, Jefferson Health, Philadelphia, Pennsylvania, USA

YOON-JEONG CHO, MD
Staff Anesthesiologist, Department of General Anesthesiology, Cleveland Clinic, Cleveland, Ohio, USA

SARAH ENSLIN, PA-C
Lead Advanced Practice Provider, Division of Gastroenterology and Hepatology, University of Rochester Medical Center, Rochester, New York, USA

JEREMY R. GLISSEN BROWN, MD
Center for Advanced Endoscopy, Division of Gastroenterology and Hepatology, Beth Israel Deaconess Medical Center, Harvard Medical School, Boston, Massachusetts, USA

MICHELLE L. HUGHES, MD
Assistant Professor, Department of Medicine, Section of Digestive Diseases, Yale School of Medicine, New Haven, Connecticut, USA

SUNGUK N. JANG, MD
Associate Director, Enterprise Endoscopy Operation, Associate Professor, Case Western Reserve University School of Medicine, Associate Section Head, Advanced Endoscopy, Department of Gastroenterology, Hepatology and Nutrition, Digestive Disease and Surgery Institute, Cleveland Clinic, Cleveland, Ohio, USA

VIVEK KAUL, MD, FACG, FASGE, AGAF
Segal-Watson Professor of Medicine, Division of Gastroenterology and Hepatology, University of Rochester Medical Center, Rochester, New York, USA

TOSSAPOL KERDSIRICHAIRAT, MD
Clinical Associate Professor of Medicine, Digestive Disease Center, Bumrungrad International Hospital, Bangkok, Thailand

ANNA M. LIPOWSKA, MD
Division of Gastroenterology and Hepatology, University of Illinois at Chicago, Chicago, Illinois, USA

GLENN D. LITTENBERG, MD, MACP, FASGE, AGAF
Chief Medical Officer, inSite Digestive Healthcare, Pasadena, California, USA

KLAUS MERGENER, MD, PhD, MBA
Affiliate Professor of Medicine, Division of Gastroenterology, University of Washington, Seattle, Washington, USA

JI SEOK PARK, MD
Department of Gastroenterology, Hepatology and Nutrition, Cleveland Clinic, Cleveland, Ohio, USA

BRET T. PETERSEN, MD
Professor of Medicine, Division of Gastroenterology and Hepatology, Mayo Clinic, Rochester, Minnesota, USA

AMANDEEP K. SHERGILL, MD, MS
Division of Gastroenterology and Hepatology, San Francisco Veterans Affairs Medical Center, University of California, San Francisco, San Francisco, California, USA

AARON J. SHIELS, MD
Rockford Gastroenterology Associates, Ltd, Rockford, Illinois, USA

EUN JI SHIN, MD, PhD
Associate Professor of Medicine, Division of Gastroenterology and Hepatology, Department of Medicine, Johns Hopkins Medical Institutions, Baltimore, Maryland, USA

EDWARD SUN, MD, MBA, FASGE
Clinical Assistant Professor, Division of Gastroenterology and Hepatology, Department of Medicine, Assistant Chief Medical Officer, Stony Brook University Hospital, Stony Brook, New York, USA

JOHN J. VARGO, MD, MPH, MASGE, AGAF, FACP, FACG, FGJES
Director, Enterprise Endoscopy Operations, Director, Endoscopic Research and Innovation, Head, Section of Advanced Endoscopy, Department of Gastroenterology, Hepatology and Nutrition, Digestive Disease and Surgery Institute, Cleveland Clinic, Associate Professor of Medicine, Cleveland Clinic Lerner College of Medicine, Case Western Reserve University, Cleveland, Ohio, USA

JOSEPH J. VICARI, MD, MBA
Rockford Gastroenterology Associates, Ltd, Rockford, Illinois, USA

Contents

Gastrointestinal (GI) endoscopy units tend to be busy environments in which numerous categories of staff provide moderately complex procedural care to high volumes of patients. The prevention of infections of both patients and staff is a never-ending endeavor for both inpatient and outpatient environments. Necessary considerations must address patient-to-staff, staff-to-patient, environmental, and device-related transmission of infection. In addition to the typical environmental and interpersonal infection risks present in all medical environments, the major concern within the endoscopy suite relates to contamination and potential transmission via reusable devices and endoscopes. Our understanding of this ever-present issue has evolved over time and has become a major focus of scrutiny in the past 5 years. This significant problem has stimulated guidance and ingenuity by regulators, investigators, and industry. Most recently, the COVID-19 pandemic of 2020 to 21 has also added significant burdens to our infection control efforts in gastrointestinal endoscopy.

Physician fatigue, also known as burnout, is a highly prevalent but often underrecognized result of workplace stressors. The consequences of burnout can include poor work–life integration, isolation, depression, and suicide. As a result, an organization may experience high physician turnover, patient safety issues, malpractice suits, and financial losses. Physicians should be encouraged to play a role in their wellness by taking mental time away from work, pursuing hobbies, attending wellness programs, and ensuring quality time with family. Ultimately, it is an organization that must acknowledge physician burnout, identify risk factors, and invest in targeted interventions to prevent this immense threat to their stability.

Optimal endoscopic operations incorporate ergonomic principles into the endoscopy environment benefiting endoscopists, endoscopy unit personnel, and patients. A high prevalence of occupational musculoskeletal injuries is well established among endoscopists and gastroenterology nurses. Ergonomics can be integrated into all facets of the endoscopy unit including scheduling, endoscopy unit design, training programs, and investment in technology. Preprocedure, intraprocedure, and postprocedure areas should aim to deliver patient safety, privacy, and comfort, while also supporting endoscopists and staff with adjustable rooms and effective work flows. Team-wide educational initiatives can improve ergonomic awareness. These strategies help mitigate risks for musculoskeletal injuries and can lead to increased productivity. The COVID-19 area brings novel challenges to endoscopy.

Endoscopy is a procedural specialty that incurs significant cost through its high usage of consumables. Thus, supply chain management and optimization in endoscopy can improve value-based care, by identifying areas of cost saving in device procurement. Creating a multidisciplinary supply chain management team, such as multidisciplinary endoscopic device committee (MEDC), suggests a way to optimize supply chain. The essential components of MEDC are physicians, clinical administration, and institutional supply chain. The physicians in the committee identify new products, define the value of products, lead the product acquisition decision-making process, and generate a practice guideline to define meaningful use of the product. The tasks of MEDC are product acquisition aligning with clinical care, review of meaningful use, and utilization of guidelines creation. In conjunction with group purchasing organization (GPO), which aggregates purchasing volume to leverage cost saving during negotiations, MEDC offers a model to optimize the endoscopy supply chain management.

 Video content accompanies this article at http://www.giendo.theclinics.com

The gastroenterology (GI) hospitalist model has improved endoscopic operations through improved interdisciplinary coordination, efficiencies introduced in endoscopy unit workflow, and increased patient access to both inpatient and outpatient GI care. The challenges and opportunities associated with a GI hospitalist model and supporting a GI hospitalist team are reviewed, especially in relation to advanced endoscopy. The roles of the GI hospitalist in endoscopy quality measurement and value-based care are also explored. Greater awareness of the GI hospitalist model and tailoring it to fit the needs of the GI practice or endoscopy unit will be key to practice sustainability and growth.

Austin L. Chiang

Social media has made a noteworthy impact in health care both in public health efforts as well as transforming how physicians connect and exchange ideas. Learning how to navigate and leverage social media across multiple platforms is becoming increasingly difficult with more platforms and features constantly being introduced. Different physicians working in the same field will have different purposes behind getting on social media, but each physician plays a different role within this social media ecosystem. This article aims to identify the common benefits of health care social media use as well as navigate the unfortunate pitfalls of social media use.

Aaron J. Shiels and Joseph J. Vicari

The future private gastroenterology practice will be a large multidisciplinary practice including a clinic, AEC, pathology services, infusion services, anesthesia services, pharmacy services, and imaging centers. Delivery of gastrointestinal (GI) services will be a team-based clinic with AEC access and improved quality of care. Competing technologies will drive practices to promote the value of colonoscopy as the best screening test for colon cancer. Artificial intelligence (AI) may significantly alter our approach to clinic and endoscopic services. The creative and intellectual capital of practice leaders will continue to define the private GI practice of the future.

John J. Vargo

The economic burden of health care in the United States continues to rise with no sign of letting up. The shift to value-based reimbursement offers a potential solution to maximize the outcome by pegging health care reimbursement to the quality of care provided. The service line concept of gastrointestinal disorders incorporates a multidisciplinary treatment model and maximizes the efficiency of patient-care giver encounters. The concept and implementation of a service line approach in endoscopy operation remain largely nascent even among large health care institutions. This article submits a multidisciplinary endoscopy operation model implemented in the author's institution as a suggestion

Tossapol Kerdsirichairat and Eun Ji Shin

Quality metrics and standardization has become critical as the Affordable Care Act mandates that the Center for Medicare and Medicaid Services change reimbursement from volume to a value-based system. While the most commonly used quality indicators are related to that of colonoscopy,

GASTROINTESTINAL ENDOSCOPY CLINICS OF NORTH AMERICA

RELATED CLINICS SERIES

Gastroenterology Clinics
(www.gastro.theclinics.com)
Clinics in Liver Disease
(www.liver.theclinics.com)

THE CLINICS ARE AVAILABLE ONLINE!
Access your subscription at:
www.theclinics.com

GASTROINTESTINAL ENDOSCOPY CLINICS
OF NORTH AMERICA

FORTHCOMING ISSUES

January 2022
Gastrointestinal Cancers and Genetic Testing
Fay Kastrinos, Editor

April 2022
Colorectal Polyps
Aasma Shaukat, Editor

July 2022
Advances in Barrett's Esophagus
Mohammad Al-Haddad, Editor

RECENT ISSUES

July 2021
Gastric Cancer
Qiin Hur, Editor

April 2021
Video Capsule Endoscopy
David R. Cave, Editor

January 2021
Advances in Barrett's Esophagus
Jacques Bergman, Editor

RELATED CLINICS SERIES

Gastroenterology Clinics
(www.gastro.theclinics.com)
Clinics in Liver Disease
(www.liver.theclinics.com)

Foreword

Endoscopic Operations: Delivering a Powerful Method with Efficiency and Quality

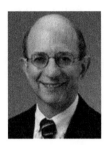

Charles J. Lightdale, MD
Consulting Editor

Dr John J. Vargo and Dr Sunguk Jang, the Editors of this issue of the *Gastrointestinal Endoscopy Clinics of North America*, are advanced endoscopists who carry out interventional procedures and study innovative methods. However, the topic they have chosen for this issue is "Optimizing Endoscopic Operations." Should this subject concern us? Absolutely! Most gastroenterologists realize that endoscopy has proven to be a highly powerful method that provides great benefit to our patients. Endoscopy keeps getting better, more accurate, more therapeutic, and more complex. How to deliver modern gastrointestinal endoscopy with efficiency and quality has become a major issue no matter where we practice. This is where endoscopic operations come into play.

I wanted to get this right, so I googled "operations," which led me to a great deal of information on how to run a business. Providing endoscopic services is a business. I distilled operations down to the process of managing a business in the most efficient manner possible. With gastrointestinal endoscopy running the gauntlet of among other things: government regulations, third-party payers, society guidelines, the emergence of the Internet and social media, a proliferation of new endoscopes and accessories, and most recently the COVID-19 pandemic, we clearly need to optimize operations. The integration of the electronic health record and of anesthesia services into the flow of endoscopy operations has been among the most difficult new challenge.

You might think that operations are a mostly back office thing of interest only to division chiefs, endoscopy directors, and the administrators of practices, hospitals, and outpatient endoscopy centers, but decisions made by operations managers will affect everyone in the endoscopy unit. Patients certainly benefit from and appreciate a well-run and efficient endoscopy service.

Gastrointest Endoscopy Clin N Am 31 (2021) xiii–xiv
https://doi.org/10.1016/j.giec.2021.07.001
1052-5157/21/© 2021 Published by Elsevier Inc.

giendo.theclinics.com

I am very grateful to Dr Vargo and Dr Jang, and to all the expert authors who contributed to this remarkable issue, which highlights an area of critical importance to current practice and to the future of gastrointestinal endoscopy.

Charles J. Lightdale, MD
Division of Digestive and Liver Diseases
Columbia University Irving Medical Center
161 Fort Washington Avenue
New York, NY 10032, USA

E-mail address:
cjl18@cumc.columbia.edu

Preface

Optimizing Endoscopic Operations

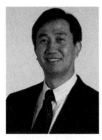   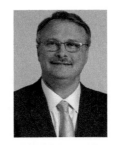

Sunguk N. Jang, MD   John J. Vargo, MD, MPH, MASGE, AGAF, FACP, FACG, FGJES
Editors

Endoscopy operations is a key part of any gastroenterology practice, be it a solo practitioner or a burgeoning health care system. A tremendous number of operational components and caregivers need to function as a cohesive and value-driven team. We have been blessed to have several experts in the field contribute to this tome. Together, these articles weave together many decades of experience and ingenuity, creating several guideposts for the reader to sample, reflect upon, and build upon their own organizational performance. Special attention was taken to discuss the power of social media, supply chain management, building a flexible and efficient organizational structure as well as approaches for the adoption of new technology and therapies.

Gastrointest Endoscopy Clin N Am 31 (2021) xv–xvi
https://doi.org/10.1016/j.giec.2021.05.013
1052-5157/21/© 2021 Published by Elsevier Inc.

In closing, we wish to thank our mentors, partners, patients, and, of course, our families for their support in this endeavor, and we welcome you, the reader, to carry on dialogs with the authors, as this work is not the end but only the beginning.

Sunguk N. Jang, MD
Section of Advanced Endoscopy
Department of Gastroenterology, Hepatology
and Nutrition
Digestive Disease and Surgery Institute
Cleveland Clinic
9500 Euclid Avenue, A-31
Cleveland, OH 44195, USA

John J. Vargo, MD, MPH, MASGE, AGAF, FACP, FACG, FGJES
Section of Advanced Endoscopy
Department of Gastroenterology, Hepatology
and Nutrition
Digestive Disease and Surgery Institute
Cleveland Clinic
9500 Euclid Avenue, A-31
Cleveland, OH 44195, USA

E-mail addresses:
jangs@ccf.org (S.N. Jang)
vargoj@ccf.org (J.J. Vargo)

Current State and Future of Infection Prevention in Endoscopy

Bret T. Petersen, MD

KEYWORDS

- Contamination • Coronavirus • Endoscopy • High level disinfection
- Infection prevention • Patients • Staff • Transmission

KEY POINTS

- Prevention of infection transmission is a never-ending endeavor in busy endoscopy departments, requiring attention to human, environmental, and equipment-related sources.
- Staff with risk of exposure to patient blood, body fluids, mucus membranes, and nonintact skin should employ "standard precautions" for hand hygiene, use of appropriate personal protective equipment, safe medication administration, and safe handling of potentially contaminated equipment.
- The risk of transmission of Coronavirus to or from clinical staff and patients undergoing endoscopy appears to be low when using diligent screening, isolation, and personal protection measures.
- The complexity of current duodenoscopes likely *precludes* reliable *absolute* reprocessing by even exemplary standard or double cycles of high-level disinfection (HLD).
- Endoscopy departments should employ diligent training, reprocessing practices, and surveillance measures to minimize risk of infection transmission resulting from insufficient endoscope reprocessing.

ENVIRONMENTAL AND INTERPERSONAL SOURCES OF INFECTION

Patients and staff are at risk of acquiring many varied infections from one another and from the procedural environment. Recent ASGE guidelines provide thorough discussions of pertinent issues and preventive practices in this regard.[1,2] In recent years, prior to the intense focus on unit practices related to COVID-19 and duodenoscope reprocessing, lapses in infection control tasks were common, as demonstrated by an audit of 68 ambulatory surgery centers sponsored by the Centers for Medicare and Medicaid Services (CMS).[3] More than two-thirds of centers had lapses and 17.6% failed to meet standards in 3 or more components of the 5 key practices surveyed. Departmental policies and procedures for infection control are mandated by

Division of Gastroenterology and Hepatology, Mayo Clinic, 201 1st Street Southwest, Rochester, MN 55905, USA
E-mail address: Petersen.bret@mayo.edu

Gastrointest Endoscopy Clin N Am 31 (2021) 625–640
https://doi.org/10.1016/j.giec.2021.05.001
1052-5157/21/© 2021 Elsevier Inc. All rights reserved.

hospital and endoscopy unit accreditation standards and the Occupational Safety and Health Administration (OHSA). Patient-facing employees in endoscopy units acquire *H. pylori* at increased rates compared to other hospital staff, but apparently not *C. difficile*. Given the risk of transmission of these and other infections to and from any individual patient is usually unknown, so-called "standard precautions," including diligent hand hygiene, use of personal protective equipment (PPE), safe medication administration practices, safe handling of potentially contaminated equipment, and cleaning of surfaces in the patient environment are all recommended for those patient interactions that carry a risk of exposure to blood, body fluids, mucus membranes, and nonintact skin.[4] The OSHA Blood-Borne Pathogens Standard (OSHA ST 29 CFR part 1910.1030)[5,6] stipulates that institutions and departmental leaders evaluate risks and educate employees regarding potential harmful exposures in the workplace (**Box 1**).

COVID-19 in the Endoscopy Unit

The COVID-19 pandemic of 2020 to 2021, caused by the spread of the SARS CoV-2 coronavirus, stimulated major changes in the entire practice of medicine, including that of GI endoscopy. As we learn more about the virus and its predominant spread by aerosols from the upper and lower respiratory tract, our unit practices for screening

---

Box 1
OSHA blood-borne pathogens standard for healthcare facilities, as applied to endoscopy facilities

1. General infection control principles should be complied with in the endoscopy unit.

2. Use of standard precautions reduces the transmission of infection from patients to endoscopy personnel.

3. Endoscopy units must have a qualified individual who directs their infection prevention plans.

4. Transmission of infection by contaminated GI endoscopes is extremely rare, and most known cases are attributable to defective endoscopes or reprocessing equipment or to lapses in performance of currently accepted endoscope reprocessing protocols.

5. Endoscopes should undergo HLD as recommended by governmental agencies and all pertinent professional organizations for the reprocessing of GI endoscopes.

6. Extensive training and documentation of training for staff involved in endoscope reprocessing is required for quality assurance and effective infection control.

7. To some extent, the efficacy of manual cleaning and HLD is operator dependent, thus highlighting the importance of process validation, extensive training, quality assurance testing of process outcome, and audits of staff performance. Staff competency should be assessed on an annual basis at the very least.

8. Particular attention should be directed toward prevention of transmission by duodenoscopes, including efforts to ensure optimal cleaning and HLD of the elevator mechanism and the biopsy and elevator wire channels.

9. In the event of reprocessing failure, the patient, the institution's designated infection control personnel, local and/or state public health agencies, the FDA, the CDC, and the manufacturers of the involved equipment should be notified immediately.

Adapted from Calderwood AH, Day LW, Muthusamy VR, and the ASGE Quality Assurance in Endoscopy Committee. ASGE guideline for infection control during GI endoscopy. Gastrointestinal Endoscopy. 87(5):1167-1179, 2018 05; with permission.

of patients and personnel, ventilation, isolation, use of personal protective gear, and environmental cleaning have all evolved.[7,8] Sagami and colleagues confirmed the significantly increased expiration of aerosols in 60 of 103 patients during (P<.001) and following (P<.001) 5-minute upper endoscopy procedures compared to preprocedure values and sham procedures (P = .006). Multivariate analysis demonstrated significant correlation between aerosol production during endoscopy and both body mass index (P = .033) and intraprocedural burping (P = .025).[9] Virions have been demonstrated in the fecal stream, and some degree of aerosol generation undoubtedly occurs, in addition to spatter and leakage of contents during colonoscopy, but this has not been as well demonstrated.[10,11] Nevertheless, use of maximal aerosol protection with N95 masks or powered air-purifying respirators (PAPRs) is necessary during all gastrointestinal endoscopy procedures during periods of known COVID prevalence in the community. Standard surgical masks always remain important for endoscopy, as several studies have confirmed pathogen deposition on endoscopists' face shields in 49% of cases and on face shields about 6 feet away in 21% of cases. Significant levels of contamination 3–4-fold beyond controls occurred in 5.6% and 3.4% of half-day procedure lists, respectively.[12] Numerous international organizations and other reports have outlined appropriate precautions for endoscopy unit operations, including considerations for preprocedure assessment of risk, intra- and postprocedure risk management, prioritization of patients, and timing of procedures.[13–18] Repici provided reassuring data regarding the risk of Coronavirus transmission to or from patients undergoing GI endoscopy in Northern Italy amidst their explosion of cases in early 2020.[19] In a single university-based tertiary hospital, careful follow-up of 851 patients identified only 1 confirmed positive case and 7 unconfirmed cases (3 COVID test-negative), and none required hospitalization. A second series reported on endoscopy unit healthcare workers from 41 of 42 regional hospitals. While 42 of 968 (4.3%) respondents tested positive for coronavirus (6 hospitalized, none in ICU), most (85.7%) presented prior to use of now standard safety measures. Most cases were clustered in 3 of the 41 centers; altogether suggesting that "GI endoscopy appears to be relatively safe for both patients and medical personnel when using adequate protective measures".[19]

PROCEDURAL INFECTIONS

Intubation of the normally soiled lumen of the upper or lower GI tract using an optimally clean instrument is generally without inherent infectious risk in immunocompetent patients. Infections after GI endoscopy typically occur as a result of: (1) translocation of microorganisms from the soiled lumen to lumens or tissues that are usually sterile, or (2) via introduction of microorganisms to the GI tract or neighboring tissues via contaminated instruments or devices. Translocation most commonly occurs during interventions that access the sterile lumen of the pancreas or biliary tree or that contaminate sterile tissues outside of the GI tract by intent or accident, via mucosal tears, puncture, or perforation. Bacteremia is most common following ERCP for obstructed ducts (18%, compared to 6.4% without obstruction), variceal sclerotherapy (up to 50% or more of cases; mean of 14.6% of cases) and esophageal stricture dilation (12% to 22%).[20] Many of these procedures warrant preventive measures or prophylactic antibiotics, particularly if persistent contamination from leakage or failed drainage can be anticipated.

The performance of endoscopic retrograde cholangiopancreatography (ERCP) in the setting of primary sclerosing cholangitis (PSC) carries a moderate risk of postprocedure cholangitis and/or intrahepatic abscess formation as a result of incomplete drainage of contaminated contrast from focally obstructed segments of the liver above persistent widespread strictures.[21] Pre- and postprocedure antibiotic prophylaxis employing an advanced penicillin, third-generation cephalosporin, or fluoroquinolone should be employed in this setting. Similarly, contrast injection into dilated bile ducts above obstructing cancers requires optimal drainage to prevent progression of local infection. When successful drainage of obstructed and contaminated ducts, by stone removal or stent placement, cannot be reliably anticipated, similar antibiotic coverage for gastrointestinal organisms of concern should be employed. The same rationale stands for extravasation of injected contrast from the biliary tree or pancreas in the setting of disrupted ducts or postoperative leaks.

Antibiotics are generally not recommended for diagnostic endoscopic ultrasonography (EUS) with or without fine-needle aspiration (FNA) for solid lesions. Data are soft and mixed for benefit of antibiotic prophylaxis prior to pancreatic or mediastinal cyst aspiration, but their use is suggested in the ASGE guidelines.[20] Many centers employ a single oral or parenteral dose.

Antibiotic prophylaxis employing first-generation cephalosporins, targeted toward cutaneous organisms, is also warranted for performance of percutaneous endoscopic gastrostomy (PEG) or jejunostomy (PEJ or PEG-J).[22] Numerous randomized trials, confirmed in a 2013 Cochrane analysis, demonstrate significant reduction in peristomal infections when cefazolin or a similarly active antibiotic is administered shortly prior to the procedure (1271 patients in 12 trials; odds ratio 0.36, 95% confidence interval .26–.50).[23] Similar prophylaxis is appropriate for most abdominal operations, including surgically assisted percutaneous transgastric ERCP in patients with Roux-en-Y gastric bypass anatomy.

Inadvertent contamination of sterile tissues, such as during overt perforation or leakage from mucosal targeted therapies, can be managed with situational administration of antibiotics. Prompt initiation of antibiotics at the first awareness of perforation or compromise of the enteric wall is advised, even intraprocedurally while initiating endoscopic efforts to repair the insult.

For so-called "third-space" procedures, including peroral endoscopic myotomy (POEM) and endoscopic submucosal dissection (ESD), many centers employ prophylactic systemic antibiotics and/or local submucosal antibiotic lavage by protocol, but limited data are available regarding their clinical benefit.

ENDOSCOPE-RELATED TRANSMISSION OF INFECTION

Transmission of exogenous microorganisms during standard esophagogastroduodenoscopy (EGD) or colonoscopy is thought to be very infrequent, but confident data on frequency of infection after general endoscopy are lacking and cases may easily go unrecognized.[1] Infrequent early reports prior to 1990 documented numerous cases of transmission of *Salmonella* during an era of cursory and nonimmersive endoscope reprocessing. Through the 1990s, occasional cases of *Pseudomonas* were reported to occur, particularly after the first ERCP of a day. Institution of thorough drying, particularly after the last case of the day, largely resolved these episodes. Outbreaks of hepatitis C have also been identified following colonoscopy and bronchoscopy in the setting of evident lapses in endoscope reprocessing and/or shared use of multidose vials for sequential patients.[24,25] Thus, for general practice of EGD and colonoscopy with straight lumen endoscopes, infection risks *appears* to be very low. Multiple national and international organizations have published guidance for practice of optimal endoscope reprocessing.[26–29] The most up-to-date iteration being the *Multisociety*

Guideline on Reprocessing Flexible GI Endoscopes and Accessories, authored by the 9 medical societies that are most intimately affiliated with the issues at hand.[30]

This presumption has been challenged by a recent report using 2014 administrative claims data from 6 states that identified emergency room visits and unplanned hospital admissions within 7 and 30 days following common outpatient procedures performed in ambulatory surgery centers (ASCs).[31] Postprocedure infection rates (within 7 days) for screening colonoscopy (1.1 per 1000 procedures), diagnostic colonoscopy (1.6/1000), and esophagogastroduodenoscopy (3.0/1000) were all significantly higher than following screening mammography (0.6/1000) but lower than following bronchoscopy (15.6/1000) or cystoscopy (4.4/1000). The rate of postendoscopy infections varied widely by more than 100-fold between individual ambulatory surgery centers and correlated with low procedure volumes, nonfreestanding ASCs, concurrent endoscopic procedures, history of recent hospitalization, and varied demographic features. These data highlight the importance of having the correct people, processes, and products in place to ensure appropriate management of endoscope reprocessing.

Several processes beyond the standard steps of *Prewash* → *Wash* → *HLD* → *Drying* have generated interest and potential utility for enhancing endoscope reprocessing outcomes. Recent and/or pending guidelines will likely call for: (1) lighted ± magnified inspection of instruments during every reprocessing cycle, (2) verification of cleaning by table-top assessment for residual biologic indicators on the endoscopes, using simple rapid swab or flush tests for adenosine triphosphate, protein, or carbohydrates,[32] (3) certification of reprocessing staff specific to care for flexible endoscopes by local or national bodies, and (4) greater specificity of the mechanism and duration of air drying between cycles and at the day's end.

Among the biologic indicators of washing efficacy, testing for residual adenosine triphosphate (ATP) is best established. It is inexpensive and requires about 5 minutes to perform, using swabs or channel flushes that are read out by a handheld device. The results do not correlate well with terminal postreprocessing cultures, but have been shown to be useful for training reprocessing personnel and monitoring performance of the washing step. In one study, Quan and colleagues demonstrated marked improvement with assessment and education of staff over 24 months of use, enabling reduction of abnormal results, indicative of insufficient washing, from 17% of cases to 2.17% of cases.[33] At present, ATP tests have not been validated or FDA cleared for use as monitoring tools during endoscope reprocessing.

Realtime video auditing of the manual washing process, which is highly dependent on the performance of individual staff members, has been shown to improve the performance of standardized maneuvers during endoscope washing in both ambulatory surgery centers[34] and tertiary advanced centers reprocessing duodenoscopes.[35] Boroscope examination of endoscopes has demonstrated a variety of nicks and scrapes to the channel lining as well as unanticipated residual droplets of water or even simethicone when drying cycles are shortened or misdirected. Routine use of boroscope exams has been proposed, but currently remains limited to investigation of damage or reduced function due to lack of specificity or meaning for many findings.[36]

DUODENOSCOPE-RELATED INFECTIONS

The most significant development in recent years pertaining to gastrointestinal endoscopy-related infections is the recognition of transmission of carbapenem-resistant Enterobacteriaceae (CRE) and other multidrug-resistant organisms (MDROs) during ERCP, first reported to occur following apparently satisfactory standard in 2014.[37] Numerous reports in the subsequent year[38,39] and others since then prompted intense investigations,[40,41] leading to the incrimination of several potential factors, primarily centered around the complexity of the common duodenoscope design[42,43] and a high risk for reprocessing failure. Given the absolute need for uninterrupted availability of duodenoscopes in clinical care, often for acute and lifesaving interventions, the path toward greater safety and absolute prevention of endoscope transmission has been ongoing but stuttering.

All duodenoscopes harbor an elevator mechanism at the distal tip for deflection of devices tangentially from the axis of the instrument. The elevator and actuating cable of standard duodenoscopes are constrained in tight spaces that are relatively inaccessible to aggressive mechanical cleaning and suboptimally exposed to cleaning and disinfecting agents that would otherwise be effective against most microorganisms. Duodenoscopes are also subject to significant stresses and wear, and thereby are at risk for greater microbial contamination and potential cleaning failure. Cleaning itself is subject to numerous failure points, largely from human factors,[44] including insufficient training, competency assessment and oversight, insufficient time allowances, excessive workload, delayed washing, and inadvertent human errors, shortcuts, or missteps that sometimes result from impractical instructions-for-use (IFU) guidance documents.[45,46]

The Food and Drug Administration (FDA) has played an important role in guiding national reprocessing practices while striving to ensure maintenance of ERCP services in the country. Most of the serial FDA guidance and safety statements are summarized in their safety statement of July, 2020.[47] In 2015, they advised renewed attention to assessment of unit reprocessing policies and performance, oversight of staff training and competency evaluations, followed by guidance to adopt one or more of several enhanced practices anticipated to improve reprocessing outcomes. Data on outcomes when employing these options are discussed below. Shortly thereafter they mandated article 522 postmarket surveillance studies of human factors and clinical outcomes in practice-based standard HLD. The 522 postmarket studies ultimately confirmed the suspected shortcomings that likely occur in general practice. Following single cycles of washing and HLD, high-concern gastrointestinal organisms were identified in 4% to 6% of endoscopes from the 3 dominant manufacturers,[39,48] with modestly lower rates in the most recent generation of instruments. Parallel contemporary results of a Dutch evaluation of postreprocessing cultures from 92% of Dutch units identified high-concern organisms in 15% of 150 duodenoscopes examined, including at least one contaminated instrument in 39% of all ERCP centers.[49]

Numerous studies have investigated the potential process enhancements advised by the FDA in 2015 and beyond, with mixed results, as briefly outlined here:

1. *Endoscope surveillance cultures:* The FDA advised use of surveillance cultures, using a subsequently proposed culture regimen developed with the Centers for Disease Control and Prevention (CDC) and the American Microbiology Society,[50] and intended specifically for surveillance rather than diagnostic purposes. This regimen has become a relative standard of practice for endoscope culturing. Published results from centers employing surveillance cultures have generally identified low but not sterile levels of enteric pathogens on reprocessed instruments. When cultured, endoscopes are advised to be held out of practice until satisfactory negative culture results return after 48 to 72 hours. A universal culture and quarantine process adopted by the Virginia Mason Clinic in Seattle[51] employs this approach for every use of a duodenoscope. Using a rigorous multipronged approach combining

universal culture and quarantine with removal and repair of serially positive endoscopes, they reduced their positive culture rate serially over time from 2.09% to 0.19% 2 years later.[52] Intermittent culture surveillance is also encouraged, and practiced by some organizations,[53] but they can be difficult and expensive to do well and without inadvertent contamination during sampling.

2. *Double cycles of HLD:* The second process enhancement proposed for consideration by the FDA is that of reprocessing duodenoscopes with double cycles of high-level disinfection. Several groups have evaluated various interpretations of this guidance. To date, results for single wash + double cycles in an automated endoscope reprocessor (AER) have not demonstrated enhanced outcomes compared to single cycles of both steps.[54,55] In contrast, using double *wash and AER* cycles, Rex and colleagues reported contamination rates similarly low to those from Virginia Mason Clinic, with only 0.32% of Olympus 160 series (1291 cultures) and 180 series (269 cultures) duodenoscopes positive for known pathogens[56] and 6% for any microorganisms.

3. *Liquid chemical sterilization (LCS):* Automated endoscope reprocessing machines employing peracetic acid (PA) (Steris, Inc. Mentor, Ohio) are FDA cleared as low-temperature "liquid chemical sterilization" technologies. Unlike other common sterilization technologies, LCS for endoscopes does not enable preservation of "terminal sterilization" in a wrapped enclosure until used at a future procedure. Once removed from the machine the device is exposed to the environment, like all instruments reprocessed with HLD. Only one recent study has compared outcomes of double wash and HLD (DHLD) (using "Rapicide PA" peracetic acid preparation in a standard AER) to LCS (peracetic acid in the Steris LCS reprocessor).[57] Altogether 978 duodenoscopes were randomly assigned to reprocessing with LCS or DHLD. Randomly performed postreprocessing culture assessment noted positive cultures in 1.9% of instruments, equally distributed between groups ($P = .8$), including only 2 high-concern organisms in each group ($P = 1.0$). No multidrug-resistant organisms were identified. The authors were unable to espouse either process over the other based upon efficacy, though times of reprocessing differences were evident.

4. *Ethylene oxide (ETO) sterilization:* A second low-temperature sterilization technology, employing ethylene oxide, has been used to terminate almost all outbreaks of duodenoscope transmission.[58] Nevertheless, ETO sterilization of duodenoscopes has undergone only limited studies, with several yielding persistence of low-concern organisms, suggesting a high likelihood of contamination during sampling, and a few demonstrating persistent organisms of concern. In a relatively small three-way study comparing single HLD versus single wash plus double HLD versus ETO sterilization, Snyder found no differences in outcome with persisting organisms in all arms of the study.[55] Case reports of failed ETO have been published, confirming the risk of failure for all but heat sterilization in the setting of insufficient washing. The most recent Multi-Society Guideline stated that use of ETO cannot be encouraged as a standard, given the limited reports and some evidence suggesting risk of failure.[30] ETO sterilization employs prolonged cycle times of up to 17 hours, due to lengthy vacuum aeration required following initial treatment. This may require significant expansion of endoscope fleets in larger practices. Ethylene oxide is highly regulated and is not available in all regions or states, due to toxicity and teratogenicity, with risk of hematologic malignancies after chronic exposure. A small table-top ETO sterilizer (EOGas4, Anderson Sterilizers, Inc., Haw River, NC) that employs much lower doses of ETO and shorter cycle times without intense negative-pressure vacuum venting has recently been

cleared for flexible endoscopes but studies from independent practice settings have not been published.

To this point in time, no single or combined processes and technologies have generated results that reliably demonstrate complete eradication of microorganisms, or even high-risk gastrointestinal organisms, from duodenoscopes and linear (therapeutic) echoendoscopes. Diligent training and processes have significantly improved surveillance culture results in several centers of excellence. Others have adopted low-temperature sterilization, often following high-level disinfection, based upon limited outcomes studies but confidence born from its use in terminating outbreaks when they have occurred.

Following return of the mandated postmarket surveillance studies of human factors and postreprocessing cultures, the FDA called for endoscopy departments to transition to duodenoscopes with removable single-use components that facilitate washing and reprocessing, or fully disposable single-use instruments.[59] In rapid sequence the 3 major manufacturers of duodenoscopes for the American market received clearance for endoscopes with disposable single-use caps (Fujinon, Olympus, and Pentax), cap and elevator (Pentax), and fully disposable duodenoscopes (AMBU and Boston Scientific) (**Box 2**).[60,61] Few data are available on the clinical use or outcomes of those instruments with removable caps. One additional technology intended to reduce transmission of infection is the ScopeSeal , a single-use device, which fits snugly over the distal tip of the duodenoscope and into the channel, effectively functioning like a condom limiting contamination onto and outward from the elevator region of the duodenoscope.[62]

Both benchtop studies and clinical results are available for the Exalt Duodenoscope, from Boston Scientific Corporation. It was deemed equivalent or better than 3 dominant reusable duodenoscopes on parameters of image quality, tip control, basket sweeping, and plastic and metal stent placement and removal.[63] Technical adjustments were then undertaken to enhance navigation and "pushability." In the first clinical study of the Exalt instrument 60 ERCPs were performed at 6 academic centers.[64] Procedures involved all ASGE complexity grades and were completed with the study duodenoscope in 58 of 60 cases. Median physician satisfaction with the instrument was 9/10, and complications typical of ERCP practice were noted in 5 patients (3 pancreatitis, 1 postsphincterotomy bleeding, 1 rehospitalized with worsening infection). In a single-center randomized trial among 98 patients, the Exalt instrument was used in 48 mostly low-complexity procedures.[65] Two patients were crossed over to reusable instruments. There were no differences in cannulation success, adverse events, or ancillary cannulation techniques. While the Exalt instrument

---

Box 2
FDA fully or partially disposable duodenoscopes, as of 7/2020

FDA-cleared single-use and fully disposable duodenoscopes:
- Ambu Innovation GmbH, Duodenoscope model aScope Duodeno
- Boston Scientific Corporation, EXALT Model D Single-Use Duodenoscope

FDA-cleared duodenoscopes with disposable end-caps and/or elevators:
- Fujifilm Corporation, Duodenoscope model ED-580XT (disposable endcap)
- Olympus Medical Systems, Duodenoscope model TJF-Q190 V (disposable endcap)
- Pentax Medical, Duodenoscope model ED34-i10 T (disposable endcap)
- Pentax Medical, Duodenoscope model ED34-i10T2 (disposable elevator and endcap)

Data from Refs.[60,61]

required fewer cannulation attempts (P = .013) it was graded "significantly worse" for image quality ($P<.001$), image stability ($P<.001$), ease of passage to the stomach (P = .047), and function of the air–water button ($P<.001$). The ability to rapidly iterate single-use devices enables continuous improvement in new device design and production. Recent clinical trials of the most current designs have been submitted for publication and larger scale studies to more clearly assess function and outcomes are underway.

New devices generate questions about function, cost, and disposal when deciding whether, when, and how to employ them in individual practices. The Exalt instrument is being marketed with inclusion of recycling and disposal services from a third party. The costs of $30,000 to $50,000 per processor and about $3000 per instrument warrants comparison to the actual cost of reprocessing existing reusable duodenoscopes. In 2019 (?), Ofstead and colleagues estimated the cost of reprocessing one endoscope to be between $114 and $281.[66] In 2020, Bang and colleagues identified a range of costs to reprocess a duodenoscope, mostly dependent on the local unit practice volume. Excluding theoretic downstream costs potentially related to cost of care for adverse events from transmitted infection, per procedure cost of use (including purchase) varied from $109 for those performing over 2000 procedures per year to $160 for units doing 500 procedures per year, and rapidly escalating to $400/case (<100 cases/y) and $800/case (<50 cases/y).[67] The 2 FDA-cleared single-use duodenoscopes were recently designated as "breakthrough devices" by the Centers for Medicare and Medicaid Services (CMS), for which CMS provides "Transitional Pass-through Codes" and add-on reimbursements to assist providers and hospitals in using newly cleared technology, while garnering several years of outcomes experience for CMS. Submission of specifically designated codes and institutional data points is required.[68,69] At present, the existing codes apply only to hospital-based care provided to Medicare-covered outpatients, but coverage for inpatient seniors is expected in the coming year.

Departmental decisions about single-use duodenoscopes, or any other technology marketed for enhanced safety and reduced risk of infection transmission, should prompt practices to assess current performance in reprocessing and their capability to improve to best practices (**Box 3**). This requires honest review of current practice, awareness beyond presumption of current outcomes using terminal cultures and potentially biological monitors on a sufficient frequency to predict performance. Many small departments aware of the cost of doing business in low volumes may consider the assessment and risk beyond reach—prompting strong interest in disposable endoscopes. For larger departments, the same data are important, but decisions may pivot around the necessity of employing the same reprocessing department, currently satisfactory outcomes, cumulative costs to buy, and environmental/consumption concerns. Situational analyses may identify specific patient risks, environments (out of unit), or timeframes (off-hours) for which selective use of single-use endoscopes is a rational starting point.[61]

WHERE IS INFECTION CONTROL IN THE ENDOSCOPY UNIT HEADED?

The pressure of growing volumes, new and more highly invasive procedures, and new infectious organisms and outbreaks will intensify the need to advance both practice and science in infection control and device reprocessing. The pandemic of 2020 to 2021 has matured our understanding of risk, prevention, and control for aerosolized viral infections and will likely push unit designs toward better aeration and space management with defined spaces for distancing of both patients and staff.

Box 3
Means to ensuring optimal reprocessing of flexible endoscopes

People
- Strive to hire and motivate a dedicated team of staff interested in adopting a professional approach to reprocessing and equipment management.
- Incorporate evidence-based reprocessing training curricula, using appropriate modalities for adult learning.
- Employ regular training updates and competency assessments
- Review and consider feasibility for adopting expectation of external credentialing of reprocessing staff.
- Ensure employment conditions are designed to retain capable staff.

Processes
- Match endoscopy calendars and throughput to capabilities of reprocessing facility and staff.
- Ensure real-time, on-site availability of concise utilitarian IFU's for cleaning and disinfection.
- Consider real-time video auditing of the manual cleaning process.
- Transition to use of only automated reprocessing equipment for sites employing manual HLD.
- Avoid use of simethicone through the accessory water channel and when required administer the lowest concentration (~0.05%) through the biopsy channel.
- Avoid delay and prolonged intervals of endoscope drying prior to washing or HLD.
- Employ ongoing per procedure and scheduled episodic assessment of endoscope structure and function.
- Employ scheduled endoscope maintenance, upgrade, parts replacements.
- Consider scheduled endoscope retirement.
- Develop capability for microbiologic assessment of duodenoscopes for scheduled surveillance and/or outbreak investigation using the FDA-proposed Duodenoscope Surveillance Sampling & Culturing regimen.
- Ensure universal 10 minute or longer direct channel drying cycles are incorporated between uses and before or during storage at day's end.
- Employ practical, validated, and outcomes-based methods for documenting performance of intermediate washing steps and outcome of high-level disinfection—for example, consider biomarkers, cultures, dryness assessments.
- Define and consider the role of patient risk profiling (eg, carbapenem-resistant Enterobacteriaceae carriers) before endoscopy and how this might impact reprocessing protocols.

Technology
- Transition duodenoscope fleet to instruments designed with single-use components.
- Consider role for single-use duodenoscopes, selectively or universally, based on local risks of transmission, known reprocessing performance, feasibility, form, function, and cost/benefit assessment.
- Submit damaged or questionable instruments for assessment and repair.
- Assess the feasibility, cost, efficacy, and impact of low-temperature sterilization technologies.
- Employ intermittent ethylene oxide sterilization for persistent culture-positive instruments and possibly following use in patients with MDRO or CRE infection or colonization.
- Follow the literature and guidance pertaining to several potentially useful technologies, including:
  - Borescope inspection of accessible endoscope channels
  - Defoaming alternatives to simethicone
  - New technologies for washing and sterilization
  - New endoscope designs and materials that enhance cleaning or sterilization efficacy

Data from Refs.[27,30,46,59,60]

Endoscope reprocessing is already advancing through regulatory and accreditation expectations, with anticipation that pending guidelines will call for certification of reprocessing staff and enhanced cleaning performance and assessment of cleaning and drying components. Recently developed nondamaging abrasive mixtures for cleaning[70] and less toxic low-temperature sterilization modalities[71] are near or initiating availability. Materials science will likely mature existing heat-tolerant endoscopes to practical widespread applications, and redesign of endoscopes can be anticipated to improve both function and ability to be fully reprocessed or sterilized. Single-use devices will undoubtedly play a role for some departments and some clinical scenarios, but they are not likely to push highly engineered reusable endoscopes from the marketplace.

TAKE-HOME MESSAGES

It is becoming clear that the complexity of endoscopes likely *precludes* reliable *absolute* reprocessing by even exemplary standard or double cycles of HLD. Current FDA guidance expects units to upgrade to new endoscope designs and more stringent guidance is likely to come. Whether society can accept an "as-low-as-reasonably-attainable" (ALARA) endpoint, like in radiation exposure or for other types of adverse outcomes, is unknown and untested in this arena. Mandated sterilization has been proposed and is viewed as our future state by many observers. New and pending technologies will undoubtedly enhance safety for ERCP using legacy reusable designs, but single-use endoscopes already provide a certain solution for the problem of infection transmission by duodenoscopes. In the meantime, it is important for all units to understand and optimize their local reprocessing performance and costs when using current instruments and reprocessing practices, while becoming familiar with the performance and costs of the alternatives before adopting them.

CLINICS CARE POINTS

- When managing an endoscopy department, ensure infection control policies are adopted, posted, communicated, and monitored, as infection outbreaks pose a high risk to the business success of the enterprise.
- Stay well informed about CDC and Gastroenterology Society guidance regarding infection precautions during the current COVID-19 pandemic.
- Establish a mechanism for identifying which patients warrant prophylactic antibiotics before endoscopic procedures in your unit and for ensuring antibiotic selection and administration or prescription pre- and postprocedure. This applies particularly to sclerosing cholangitis, as failure to cover ERCP interventions in this patient group risks development of cholangitis or liver abscesses.
- Develop a means for assigning time stamps to intervals critical to endoscope reprocessing to ensure timely completion of bedside prewash and subsequent washing steps, the latter within 1 hour of extubation, to avoid premature drying and fixation of contaminating microorganisms.
- Ensure adoption of a dedicated drying step after high-level disinfection, employing either forced filtered air through the endoscope channels for a minimum of 10 minutes or use of a drying cabinet for storage. Note, drying with a manually operated forced-air gun directed to the exterior and channels will not suffice, as interior drying is insufficient with this approach.
- Ensure use of advised elevator manipulation up and down during washing maneuvers and positioning in a midrange position during automated high-level disinfection, to reduce the risk of retained contaminants in the elevator recess.

- Develop or adopt unit-specific policies for maximum "hang-time" of endoscopes, to ensure reprocessing is performed within an appropriate timeframe prior to use—generally 7, 10, 14, or 21 days.
- Consider and adopt one or more mechanisms for surveillance assurance of adequate washing and/or overall reprocessing, including possible use of biomarkers after washing steps (ATP, etc.) or culture surveillance after full cycles of high-level disinfection.
- Adopt practice of routine inspection of each endoscope for defects or damage, including with each washing cycle and intermittent in-depth assessment.

DISCLOSURE

Olympus America—Consultant, Boston Scientific—Investigator, Ambu—Investigator.

REFERENCES

1. Calderwood AH, Day LW, Muthusamy VR. and the ASGE Quality Assurance in Endoscopy Committee. ASGE guideline for infection control during GI endoscopy. Gastrointest Endosc 2018;87(5):1167–79.
2. Calderwood AH, Chapman FJ, Cohen J. and the ASGE Ensuring Safety in the Gastrointestinal Endoscopy Unit Task Force. Guidelines for safety in the gastrointestinal endoscopy unit. Gastrointest Endosc 2014;79(3):363–72.
3. Schaefer MK, Jhung M, Dahl M, et al. Infection control assessment of ambulatory surgical centers. JAMA 2010;303:2273–9.
4. Guide to infection prevention for outpatient settings: Minimum expectations for safe care. Available at: https://www.cdc.gov/infectioncontrol/pdf/Fillable-Outpatient-Checklist_508.pdf. Accessed February 10, 2021.
5. Occupational exposure to bloodborne pathogens–OSHA. Final rule. Fed Regist 1991;56:64004–182.
6. Occupational exposure to bloodborne pathogens; needlestick and other sharps injuries; final rule. Occupational Safety and Health Administration (OSHA), Department of Labor. Final rule; request for comment on the information collection (paperwork) requirements. Fed Regist 2001;66:5318–25.
7. Tian Y, Rong L, Nian W, et al. Review article: gastrointestinal features in COVID-19 and the possibility of faecal transmission. Aliment Pharmacol Ther 2020;51: 843–51.
8. Hussain A, Singhal T, EL-Hasani S. Extent of infectious SARS-CoV-2 aerosolisation as a result of oesophago-gastroduodenoscopy or colonoscopy. Br J Hosp Med 2020. https://doi.org/10.12968/hmed.2020.0348.
9. Sagami R, Nishikiori H, Sato T, et al. Aerosols produced by upper gastrointestinal endoscopy: a quantitative evaluation. Am J Gastroenterol 2021;116(1):202–5.
10. Cheung KS, Hung IFN, Chan PPY, et al. Gastrointestinal manifestations of SARS-CoV-2 infection and virus load in fecal samples from a hong kong cohort: systematic review and meta-analysis. Gastroenterology 2020;159(1):81–95.
11. Chen C, Gao G, Xu Y, et al. SARS-CoV-2-positive sputum and faeces after conversion of pharyngeal samples in patients with COVID-19. Ann Intern Med 2020; 172(12):832–4.
12. Johnston ER, Habib-Bein N, Dueker JM, et al. Risk of bacterial exposure to the endoscopist's face during endoscopy. Gastrointest Endosc 2019;89(4):818–24.
13. Covid 19 updates for members. Available at: https://www.asge.org/home/resources/key-resources/covid-19-asge-updates-for-members/asge-covid-19-

frequently-asked-questions#how-should-rooms-be-cleaned-at-the-end-of-the-day-if-a-high-risk-patient-has-had-endoscopy-in-the-room. Accessed February 15, 2021.

14. Guda NM, Emura F, Reddy DN, et al. Recommendations for the Operation of Endoscopy Centers in the setting of the COVID-19 pandemic - World Endoscopy Organization guidance document. Dig Endosc 2020;32(6):844–50.
15. Chiu PWY, Ng SC, Inoue H, et al. Practice of endoscopy during COVID-19 pandemic: Position statements of the Asian Pacific Society for Digestive Endoscopy (APSDE-COVID statements). Gut 2020;69:991–6.
16. Gralnek IM, Hassan C, Beilenhoff U, et al. ESGE and ESGENA Position Statement on gastrointestinal endoscopy and the COVID-19 pandemic 2020. Available at: https://www.esge.com/esge-and-esgena-position-statement-on-gastrointestinal-endoscopy-and-the-covid-19-pandemic/. Accessed February 15, 2021.
17. Lui RN, Wong SH, Sanchez-Luna SA, et al. Overview of guidance for endoscopy during the coronavirus disease 2019 (COVID-19) pandemic. J Gastroenterol Hepatol 2020;35:749–59.
18. Repici A, Maselli R, Colombo M, et al. Coronavirus (COVID-19) outbreak: what the department of endoscopy should know. 2020. Gastrointest Endosc 2020;92(1):192–7.
19. Repici A, Aragona G, Cengia G, et al, ITALIAN GI-COVID19 Working Group. Low risk of COVID-19 transmission in GI endoscopy. Gut 2020;69(11):1925–7.
20. Khashab MA, Chithadi K, Acosta RD, the ASGE Standards of Practice Committee. Antibiotic prophylaxis for GI endoscopy. Gastrointest Endosc 2015;81(1):81–9.
21. Bangarulingam SY, Gossard A, Petersen BT, et al. Complications of endoscopic retrograde cholangiopancreatography in primary sclerosing cholangitis. Am J Gastroenterol 2009;104(4):855–60.
22. Jain NK, Larson DE, Schroder KW, et al. Antibiotic prophylaxis for percutaneous endoscopic gastrostomy. Ann Intern Med 1987;107(6):824-8.
23. Lipp A, Lusardi G. Systemic antimicrobial prophylaxis for percutaneous endoscopic gastrostomy. Cochrane Database Syst Rev 2013;(11):CD005571.
24. Bronowicki JP, Venard V, Botte C, et al. Patient-to-patient transmission of hepatitis C virus during colonoscopy. N Engl J Med 1997;337:237–40.
25. Fischer GE, Schaefer MK, Labus BJ, et al. Hepatitis C virus infections from unsafe injection practices at an endoscopy clinic in Las Vegas, Nevada, 2007-2008. Clin Infect Dis 2010;51(3):267–73.
26. Essential Elements of a Reprocessing Program for Flexible Endoscopes – Recommendations of the HICPAC. Available at: https://www.cdc.gov/hicpac/pdf/flexible-endoscope-reprocessing.pdf. Accessed February 26, 2021.
27. Petersen BT, Cohen J, Hambrick RD 3rd, et al, Reprocessing Guideline Task Force. Multisociety guideline on reprocessing flexible GI endoscopes: 2016 update. Gastrointest Endosc 2017;85:282–94.
28. Herrin A, Loyola M, Bocian S, et al. SGNA Practice Committee 2015-16. Standards of infection prevention in reprocessing flexible gastrointestinal endoscopes. Gastroenterol Nurs 2016;39(5):404–18.
29. Beilenhoff U, Biering H, Blum R, et al. Reprocessing of flexible endoscopes and endoscopic accessories used in gastrointestinal endoscopy: Position Statement of the European Society of Gastrointestinal Endoscopy (ESGE) and European Society of Gastroenterology Nurses and Associates (ESGENA) - Update 2018. Endoscopy 2018;50:1205–34.

30. Day LW, Muthusamy VR, Collins J, et al. Multisociety Guideline on Reprocessing Flexible GI Endoscopes and Accessories. Gastrointest Endosc 2021;93(1): 11–33.e6.

31. Wang P, Xu T, Ngamruengphong S, et al. Rates of infection after colonoscopy and esophagogastroduodenoscopy in ambulatory surgery centres in the USA. Gut 2018;67:1626–36.

32. ASGE Technology Committee. Biologic Indicators. Gastrointest Endosc 2014; 80(3):369–72.

33. Quan E, Mahmood R, Naik A, et al. Use of adenosine triphosphate to audit reprocessing of flexible endoscopes with an elevator mechanism. Am J Infect Control 2018;46:1272–7.

34. Lan G, Tsistrakis S, Bernstein BB. Remote Video Auditing With Feedback in an Ambulatory Endoscopy Suite: Impact on Compliance With Endoscope Cleaning Protocols Gastrointestinal. Endoscopy 2017;85(5S):AB66.

35. Raphael KL, McNoble E, Goldbeck J, et al. Remote video auditing in the endoscopy unit for evaluation of duodenoscope reprocessing in a tertiary care center. Endoscopy 2020;52(10):864–70.

36. Visrodia K, Petersen BT. Borescope examination: Is there value in visual assessment of endoscope channels? Gastrointest Endosc 2018;88(4):620–3.

37. Epstein L, Hunter JC, Arwady MA, et al. New Delhi metallo-betalactamase-producing carbapenem-resistant Escherichia coli associated with exposure to duodenoscopes. JAMA 2014;312:1447–55.

38. Wendorf KA, Kay M, Baliga C, et al. Endoscopic Retrograde Cholangiopancreatography-Associated AmpC Escherichia coli Outbreak. Infect Control Hosp Epidemiol 2015;36:634–42.

39. Petersen BT. Duodenoscope reprocessing: risk and options coming into view. Gastrointest Endosc 2015;82:484–7.

40. United States Senate – Health, Education, Labor and Pensions Committee. Patty Murray, Ranking Member. Preventable Tragedies: Superbugs and How Ineffective Monitoring of Medical Device Safety Fails Patients. Available at: https://www.help.senate.gov/imo/media/doc/Duodenoscope%20Investigation%20FINAL%20Report.pdf. Accessed February 15, 2021.

41. Verfaillie CJ, Bruno MJ, Voor in 't holt AF, et al. Withdrawal of a novel-design duodenoscope ends outbreak of a VIM-2-producing Pseudomonas aeruginosa. Endoscopy 2015;47:502.

42. Petersen KJ, Ginsberg GG. AGA Clinical Practice Commentary: Infection Using ERCP Endoscopes. Gastroenterology 2016;151:46–50.

43. Ofstead CL, Hopkins KM, Buro BL, et al. State of the Science Review: Challenges in achieving effective high-level disinfection in endoscope reprocessing. Am J Infect Control 2020;48:309–15.

44. Ofstead CL, Wetzler HP, Snyder AK, et al. Endoscope reprocessing methods: a prospective study on the impact of human factors and automation. Gastroenterol Nurs 2010;33:304–11.

45. Available at: https://www.accessdata.fda.gov/scripts/cdrh/cfdocs/cfPMA/pss.cfm?t_id=354&c_id=3692. Accessed February 15, 2021.

46. Day LW, Kwok K, Visrodia K, et al. American Society for Gastrointestinal Endoscopy Infection Control Summit: updates, challenges, and the future of infection control in GI endoscopy. Gastrointest Endosc 2020;91(1):1–10.

47. FDA Safety Communication of 7/24/20. Available at: https://www.fda.gov/medical-devices/safety-communications/fda-recommending-transition-duodenoscopes-

innovative-designs-enhance-safety-fda-safety-communication#reprocessing. Accessed February 15, 2021.

48. FDA 522 Data reports – Olympus Company. Available at: https://www. accessdata.fda.gov/scripts/cdrh/cfdocs/cfPMA/pss.cfm?t_id=354&c_id=3726. Accessed February 15, 2021.

49. Rauwers AW, Voor In't Holt AF, Buijs JG, et al. High prevalence rate of digestive tract bacteria in duodenoscopes: a nationwide study. Gut 2018;67(9):1637–45.

50. Duodenoscope Surveillance Sampling and Culturing. Available at: https://www. fda.gov/media/111081/download. Accessed February 15, 2021.

51. Ross AS, Baliga C, Verma P, et al. A quarantine process for the resolution of duodenoscope-associated transmission of multidrug resistant *Escherichia coli*. Gastrointest Endosc 2015;82:477–83.

52. Higa JT, Choe J, Tombs D, et al. Optimizing duodenoscope reprocessing: rigorous assessment of a culture and quarantine protocol. Gastrointest Endosc 2018;88(2):223–9.

53. Thaker AM, Muthusamy VR, Sedarat A, et al. Duodenoscope reprocessing practice patterns in U.S. endoscopy centers: a survey study. Gastrointest Endosc 2018;88(2):316–22.e2.

54. Bartles RL, Leggett JE, Hove S, et al. A randomized trial of single versus double high-level disinfection of duodenoscopes and linear echoendoscopes using standard automated reprocessing. Gastrointest Endosc 2018;88(2):306–13.

55. Snyder GM, Wright SB, Smithey A, et al. Randomized comparison of 3 high-level disinfection and sterilization procedures for duodenoscopes. Gastroenterology 2017;153:1018–25.

56. Rex DK, Sieber M, Lehman GA, et al. A double-reprocessing high-level disinfection protocol does not eliminate positive cultures from the elevators of duodenoscopes. Endoscopy 2018;50:588–96.

57. Gromski MA, Sieber MS, Sherman S, et al. Double high-level disinfection versus liquid chemical sterilization for reprocessing of duodenoscopes used for ERCP: a prospective randomized study. Gastrointest Endosc 2021;93(4):927–31.

58. Muscarella LF. Use of ethylene-oxide gas sterilization to terminate multidrug-resistant bacterial outbreaks linked to duodenoscopes. BMJ Open Gastroenterol 2019;6(1):e000282.

59. FDA recommends health care facilities and manufacturers begin transitioning to duodenoscopes with disposable components to reduce risk of patient infection (August 19, 2019). Available at: https://www.fda.gov/news-events/press-announcements/ fda-recommends-health-care-facilities-and-manufacturers-begin-transitioning-duodenoscopes-disposable. Accessed February 15, 2021.

60. FDA cleared Duodenoscopes with enhanced designs incorporating removable components. Available at: https://www.fda.gov/medical-devices/safety-communications/ fda-recommending-transition-duodenoscopes-innovative-designs-enhance-safety-fda-safety-communication#reprocessing. Accessed February 15, 2021.

61. Trindade AJ, Copland A, Bhatt A, et al, ASGE Technology Committee. Single use duodenoscopes and duodenoscopes with disposable end caps. Gastrointest Endosc 2021;93(5):997–1005.

62. Pasricha PJ, Miller S, Carter F, et al. Novel and effective disposable device that provides 2-way protection to the duodenoscope from microbial contamination. Gastrointest Endosc 2020;92(1):199–208.

63. Ross AS, Bruno MJ, Kozarek RA, et al. Novel single-use duodenoscope compared with 3 models of reusable duodenoscopes for ERCP: a randomized bench-model comparison. Gastrointest Endosc 2020 Feb;91(2):396–403.

64. Muthusamy VR, Marco J, Bruno MJ, et al. Clinical Evaluation of a Single-Use Duodenoscope for Endoscopic Retrograde Cholangiopancreatography. Clin Gastroenterol Hepatol 2020;18:2108–17.
65. Bang JY, Hawes R, Varadarajulu S. Equivalent performance of single-use and reusable duodenoscopes in a randomised trial. Gut 2021;70(5):838–44.
66. Ofstead CL, Quick MR, Eiland JE, et al. A GLIMPSE AT THE TRUE COST OF REPROCESSING ENDOSCOPES: RESULTS OF A PILOT PROJECT. IAHSCM Communique. Available at: https://www.bostonscientific.com/content/dam/bostonscientific/uro-wh/portfolio-group/LithoVue/pdfs/Sterilization-Resource-Handout.pdfl. Accessed June 23, 2021.
67. Bang JY, Sutton B, Hawes R, et al. Concept of disposable duodenoscope: at what cost? Gut 2019;68:1915–7.
68. What Does the New Pass-Through Payment Mean for the Single-Use Duodenoscope? American Society for Gastrointestinal Endoscopy. Available at: https://www.asge.org/docs/default-source/default-document-library/new-pass-through-code–final.pdf. Accessed February 25, 2021.
69. Boston Scientific. Medicare Transitional Pass-Through Payment Applicable to EXALT™ Model D Single Use Duodenoscope. Available at: https://www.bostonscientific.com/content/dam/bostonscientific/Reimbursement/Gastroenterology/pdf/TPT_Customer_Billing_Guide.pdf. Accessed February 25, 2021.
70. Available at: www.novaflux.com. Accessed February 15, 2021.
71. Molloy-Simard V, Lemyre J, Martel K, et al. Elevating the standard of endoscope processing: Terminal sterilization of duodenoscopes using a hydrogen peroxide–ozone sterilizer. Am J Infect Control 2019;47(3):243–50.

Managing Physician Fatigue

Asyia Ahmad, MD, MPH*

KEYWORDS

• Physician fatigue • Physician burnout • Work–life integration • Work-related stress

KEY POINTS

• Physician fatigue, also known as burnout, is a direct result of workplace stressors which include administrative hassles, work-flow inefficiencies, work hour burdens, and ineffective leadership.
• Physician burnout is often underrecognized by both the physician and his/her organization and can lead to depression, suicide, and negatively impacts work–life balance.
• Organizations must acknowledge physician burnout as a threat to their financial stability requiring ongoing focused intervention.

BACKGROUND

Physician fatigue, often referred to as burnout, was first coined by Herbert Freudenberger, a German-born American psychologist known for his observations at a drug abuse clinic in New York City in the 1970s. It was there that he noticed fatigue, irritability, cynicism, isolation, and headaches in staff who worked with drug abuse addicts and ironically coined the phrase "burnout." He ultimately defined burnout as excessive workplace demands on an individual's energy, strength, and resources.[1] The work by social psychologist Christina Maslach in the late 1970s expanded on Freudenberger's concept of burnout. Maslach focused on human service professionals and noted additional consequences of burnout including low staff morale, absenteeism, high job turnover, marital and family issues, and drug abuse.[2] She eventually created the Maslach Burnout Index (MBI), a 25-question validated tool ascertaining burnout in terms of emotional exhaustion, depersonalization, and personal accomplishment.[3] This screening tool has been modified over the last 4 decades but remains one of the most utilized tools for assessing burnout today.

The work described by both Freudenberger and Maslach has been largely underrecognized until the last decade. In fact, it was only in 2016 that occupational or job burnout was included in the International Category of Diseases (ICD) as a billable code. Occupational burnout or job burnout is defined by ICD-10 as a type of

Division of Gastroenterology, Drexel University College of Medicine/Tower Health Medical Group, Philadelphia, PA, USA
* The Pavilion at Doylestown Hospital, 599 W. State Street, Suite 200, Doylestown, PA 18901, USA
E-mail address: Asyiaahmad4@gmail.com

Gastrointest Endoscopy Clin N Am 31 (2021) 641–653
https://doi.org/10.1016/j.giec.2021.05.002
1052-5157/21/© 2021 Elsevier Inc. All rights reserved.

psychological stress categorized by exhaustion, lack of enthusiasm and motivation, feelings of ineffectiveness, frustration, or cynicism and, as a result, reduced efficacy within the workplace. The ICD-11 definition destigmatizes burnout by clarifying it as an occupational phenomenon not a medical or psychiatric condition.[4]

PHYSICIAN BURNOUT RATE

Although burnout has been highly linked to all human services professionals, physician burnout has been especially devastating and begins as early as medical school. Interestingly, students entering medical school have higher mental health profiles than their counterparts in other fields; however, this trend rapidly reverses within 2 years after matriculation.[5] Medical trainees can also experience immense fatigue. In fact, 60% of medical residents and fellows in training satisfy criteria for burnout, which is significantly higher than age-matched controls.[6] The loss of community secondary to changing rotations and care teams contributes to isolation and burnout during the training years.[7]

Physician fatigue after the training years has been extensively studied. A systematic review of 182 studies reported a physician burnout rate of between 0% to 82% with differences due to study size, design, and measurement tools.[8] Physician burnout is likely closer to 46%, which is significantly elevated above other professions. Specialties such as emergency medicine, family medicine, and internal medicine ranked highest on the burnout scale.[9] In a 2013 survey, gastroenterology rated 17th out of 24th in burnout rates with emergency medicine and critical care rating at the top.[10] Burnout rates in gastroenterologists range from 34% to 50%,[11] with early-career gastroenterologists revealing the highest rates.[12] Early-career burnout is prevalent in other procedure-related disciplines such as surgery,[13] where unique concerns with procedural competence, reimbursement, procedure-related adverse outcomes, and missed cancers are common. Similarly, early-career interventional endoscopists have higher burnout scores than noninterventionalists. Trends toward working in academic institutions with more complex patients, longer work hours, and involvement in high-risk procedures are responsible for this finding.[14]

CONSEQUENCES OF BURNOUT

Consequences of burnout include both depression and suicide. A large study reported that 37.8% of physicians are depressed as measured by a standardized, validated questionnaire.[9] The combination of depression and burnout can lead to suicidal ideation and suicide. A meta-analysis found that physician suicide is 30 times that of the general population in men and 130 times that of the general population in women.[15] Although men are more likely to die by suicide than women in the general population, this discrepancy disappears as early as medical school, where the rates of suicide escalate in women. Higher rates of psychiatric disorders in physicians coupled with drug and alcohol abuse are associated with physician suicide. Physicians are more likely to be successful with suicide attempts, which is related to their access and familiarity with lethal drugs.[16] Physicians are more likely to die by poisoning than by any other method, and over half have accessed the poisons at work.[17] Job stressors, debt, social isolation, feelings of incompetence, perfectionism, and familiarity with death at work predispose physicians to suicide.[18]

Inability to succeed in work–life integration is known to cause emotional and mental instability in physicians. Work–life integration is the productive and supportive interaction between one's professional and personal lives. Although physicians are generally satisfied with their careers, less than 50% are satisfied with their work–life integration. Control over their schedule and number of hours worked are the greatest predictors of work–life satisfaction regardless of age, gender, or specialty.[19] Between 2011 and 2014, work–life integration appeared to diminish overall for physicians, even after adjusting for hours worked, gender, age, and relationship status. Only 36% of physicians felt that their professional career allowed adequate time for their personal or home life, which was significantly lower than the general workforce. Of the medicine specialties, only obstetricians and gynecologists saw an improvement in work–life integration with all other physicians reporting diminishing quality. Not unexpectedly, surgical and medical subspecialties consistently rated their work–life integration below the overall physician mean.[20]

Poor work–life integration has a negative impact on both the physician and their family. A national study of US physician partners found that partners reported that their physician partner often came home tired, irritable, or preoccupied with work. On a multivariant analysis, the number of nights on call per week significantly correlated with home life dissatisfaction regardless of hours of work during the day, type of practice, or specialty.[21] Divorce is also a potential result of burnout, with women physicians 1.5 times more likely to divorce than men physicians. Women who work 40 or more hours per week were more likely to divorce than women who worked less than 40 hours per week. Interestingly, this trend was opposite in men.[22] Women physicians are also more likely to believe that their professional life negatively impacts their children. The number of hours worked per week negatively impacted parental satisfaction, with each extra hour worked decreasing satisfaction by 1%. Women who were married or worked in an academic setting admit to higher satisfaction with their parental relationships than their counterparts.[23]

RISK FACTORS FOR BURNOUT

Administrative burdens are one of the top reasons for physician burnout and fatigue. Administrative burdens include usage of electronic health records, insurance authorization, claims, and billing. Other often overlooked technologic burdens include mandatory Internet trainings, malfunctioning computers, excessive patient- and staff-generated electronic messages, and unnecessary emails.[24] The 2009 Health Information Technology for Economic and Clinical Health Act provided federal incentives for the implementation of electronic medical records. This rapid change led to increased demands and time for documentation. In fact, one large study of physicians found that for every 1 hour of direct patient care, primary care physicians spent an additional 1.4 hours on electronic health documentation.[25] In addition to increased time demands, difficulty in usability has contributed to physician dissatisfaction. A study of over 5000 physicians reported that favorable Electronic Health Record usability was significantly related to lower burnout scores regardless of age, gender, type of practice, or hours worked.[26]

Ineffective leadership can directly compromise the culture and stability of an organization and lead to emotional exhaustion and stress within the work unit, increase employee turnover, and engender unprofessional behaviors. In fact, over 75% of people rate their direct leader as the most significant source of stress at work.[27] Two types of leaders can destabilize an organization. The first is the destructive leader who has bullying behaviors. The other is the laissez-faire or passive leader who avoids stressful situations which require swift action. Passive leadership is often underrecognized even though it can lead to psychological work fatigue, poor work attitude, and work role conflict.[28] Physician leaders serve as unique and important liaisons in many organizations. One study of close to 4000 physicians evaluated immediate physician leaders on 12 measurable and actionable qualities including ability to inform, engage, inspire, develop, and recognize other physicians. High composite leadership scores led to a 3.3% lower risk for physician burnout and a 9.9% likelihood for satisfaction within the work unit.[29]

Another underappreciated risk factor is medical errors and malpractice lawsuits. Physicians who face lawsuits may feel ashamed, isolated, depressed, or suicidal. In addition, inadvertent medical errors may lead to future defensive practices and overwhelming long-term emotional exhaustion. Overall, physicians who practice in procedural specialties, such as gastroenterology, face higher risks for malpractice than physicians that do not.[30]

THE COST OF BURNOUT TO AN ORGANIZATION

A burned-out physician is three times as likely to leave their position within 2 years than a physician that is not burned out after controlling for underlying depression, sleep disorders, work hours, and anxiety. The cost to recruit and replace a physician has been quantified at a staggering $268,000 to $957,000, and varies based on specialty and experience.[31] In fact, the estimated losses from decreased productivity and burnout are reported to be around 4.6 billion dollars every year or 7600 dollars per physician per year.[32] Organizations may also face patient safety issues as medical errors are reported to be higher in physicians that are burned out. In fact, self-reported medical errors and lower quality of care were significantly higher in physicians with burnout. Overall, physician burnout led to an increased risk of patient safety incidents, poorer quality of care, and lower patient satisfaction scores.[33] Patients under the care of physicians with burnout are less likely to adhere to recommendations and report poor relationships with their provider.[34] Medical errors coupled to poor patient satisfaction can raise the risk of malpractice suits within an organization.

IDENTIFYING BURNOUT IN PHYSICIANS

Physician burnout can lead to medical errors, poor patient satisfaction, decreased quality of care, and turnover, therefore it is imperative that at-risk physicians are identified. Physicians often lack insight and awareness of personal issues with fatigue and burnout. In fact, a large study showed that over 70% of surgeons with Physician Wellness Index scores at the lowest 30%, believed they were at or above national physician norms.[35] Furthermore, physicians may not be willing to acknowledge any struggles they are facing for fear of professional consequences including issues with credentialing and licensing.

Since its creation, the MBI has been utilized extensively as the best validated measure of physician burnout. The MBI is a dichotomous scale with no set cutoff value for physician burnout. Previous studies have utilized it haphazardly with omission of subcategories such as personal accomplishment. Inclusion of important individual factors including cynicism and workplace factors are not included in the MBI.[36] Lastly, the MBI does not evaluate the impact burnout has on an organization.

Various scales have been created since the implementation of the MBI, and the Physician Wellbeing Index is perhaps the best global substitute for the MBI. This brief 7-question survey evaluates not only fatigue and emotional distress but also assesses a person's career satisfaction and job performance. This scale is attractive to organizations as it can assess individual burnout as well as the financial impact on an organization.[3] Another simple screening tool is a 2-question inquiry focused on emotional exhaustion and depersonalization. Physicians are deemed burned out if they answer yes to 2 focused questions that ask if an individual feels burned out by their work, and if they have become callous toward people since taking the job.[37]

COMBATING PHYSICIAN BURNOUT

Physician wellbeing has become a top priority of many organizations. In 2017, both the National Academy of Science[38] and CEOs of major healthcare organizations[39] separately set forth to uncover the instigating factors threatening physician wellbeing. Through these focused groups, over 80 individual variables that lead to physician burnout were identified. Prioritizing factors have become an increasing challenge as an organization may have multiple concurrent primary risk factors for physician burnout. In addition, each work unit may face different priority issues, leading to difficulty in creating a universal strategy to deal with the crisis. Lastly, the inability of organizational leaders to uncover the true underlying causes of burnout may lead to faulty interventions that only exacerbate the ongoing problem.[40]

A large systemic review evaluating controlled interventions for combating physician burnout found that organizational directed interventions resulted in more positive results than individual measures.[41] This is not surprising as physicians must have insight into their own fatigue and mental wellbeing to utilize and benefit from self-directed interventions. As a result, studies evaluating burnout outcomes utilizing self-directed measures may be inherently biased by self-selection. Although important, self-directed interventions cannot address or change work-driven stresses and should serve as a complement to a global strategy.

ORGANIZATIONAL STRATEGIES FOR REDUCING BURNOUT

Work environment and structure can greatly impact a physician's wellbeing and must be critically evaluated to prevent burnout. In the multicenter Healthy Workplace Study, primary care physicians were significantly less likely to be stressed, had lower burnout scores, and were less likely to want to leave their job with interventions focused on offloading nonessential physician tasks such as faxing and basic data entry into the EMR, pairing medical assistants with physicians, ensuring adequate number of staff, and increasing office visit time. Interestingly, scheduling physician meetings to discuss work–life issues and difficult patient cases did not have as big an effect.[42] Other organizational opportunities include ensuring adequate office space and needed resources to successfully complete daily tasks. Encouraging cross-training of staff and utilizing scribes can also decrease physician fatigue.

Work hour demands play a large role in physician burnout. Interventions that have altered call schedules and instituted flexible work hours have overwhelmingly positive results. For example, intensivists who worked day shifts within a week but were then given nights free of call were significantly less fatigued than those that worked during the day with simultaneous nighttime call. Shorter inpatient rotations and time off from work during the weekday also significantly improved physician fatigue. Flexible work schedules have been shown to significantly improve physician wellbeing. In a large prospective randomized trial, surgical resident physicians overwhelmingly chose flexible work hours with longer but fewer shifts. Flexible schedules were shown to improve patient care, personal wellbeing, and educational value.[43] This theme should be utilized in all institutions by considering staggered early or late hours or utilizing longer 4-day work weeks. These strategies also appeal to patients as well as staff who often face similar challenges with work–life integration. Organizations should reevaluate salary compensation and should eliminate incentives based solely around RVU (relative value units) generation. Allowing physicians to engage in work that is deemed meaningful for them for at least 20% of the time can also significantly decrease burnout.[44]

Improving leadership effectiveness is another crucial facet to reducing emotional exhaustion. Leaders serve as the agent of an organization's values and leaders with ethical characteristics directly lead to less emotional exhaustion and greater job satisfaction among their employees.[27] Two-way communication with employees, adequate resources, and development of a nonintimidating, moral environment have been shown to be effective in a study of frontline workers.[45] In circumstances where stress is induced by the leader, evaluating leaders or rotating leadership on a consistent basis are strategies that can be used. Investing in leadership training should be a priority. Currently there are no standardized course requirements for obtaining a leadership role. One could easily argue that leadership training programs should be required starting as early as medical school, as physicians often lead work units impacting students, residents, and medical staff, groups also at high risk for professional burnout.

Organizations should consider investing in a professional coach as a powerful resource for both leaders and physicians. A coach utilizes active listening to ask powerful questions that lead to a person's self-awareness. A coach can also motivate individuals to take effective steps to reach resolutions and navigate work stressors. In medicine, coaches can perhaps be most useful in cases where physician leaders are asked to address a difficult and stressful situation that needs careful resolution such as harassment involving coworkers, staff, or patients. Coaches can also be useful in guiding specific physicians who are overly fatigued or have maladapted coping styles. In a study of 88 physicians, emotional exhaustion scores and overall burnout significantly declined in the group of physicians who received 6 coaching sessions compared to the group that did not.[46] A large study of gastroenterologists found that physician fatigue is likely exacerbated in physicians that utilize emotion-focused coping, which includes self-blame, denial, venting, and distraction. Coaches may help motivate individuals to approach stress with active problem-focused methods, which have been shown to be more effective and decrease burnout rates.[47]

Creative utilization of available resources and support systems can curb physician fatigue. The creation of safe zones for physician gatherings such as lounges or break rooms can naturally create camaraderie and a sense of community. Discussions of stressful patient care issues and personal challenges can decrease loneliness and isolation. Peer support groups are a more structured means of connecting physicians who may share emotional or traumatic experiences such as an inadvertent medical error or patient death. Mentorship is also critical for career development and may alleviate insecurities surrounding competence which are often seen in early-career physicians. In fact, physicians that engage in peer support groups or have mentors have higher career satisfaction and experience less burnout.[48]

INDIVIDUAL STRATEGIES TO PREVENT BURNOUT

Individual strategies for physician's wellbeing need to be actively practiced. One of the basic strategies is to take mental time away from work by shutting off electronic devices and phones, being present for important family time, and engaging in hobbies and personal fitness.[49] In fact, surgeons that saw their primary care physician in the last year, engaged in aerobic exercise, and participated in wellness programs were found to have significantly higher physical and quality-of-life scores than surgeons that did not.[50] Utilizing outside help for work around the home and with childcare can free up needed time. Engaging in self-directed mindfulness programs can be highly successful for relieving stress. On the other hand, organizational-directed participation may not be attended by physicians most in need of the services.[51] Stress reduction and self-care workshops, exercise programs, and mindfulness retreats have all reported to improve burnout. Actively engaging leadership to discuss work duties and schedules may also be useful in preventing fatigue and burnout. Learning to say no to extra work that has no personal benefit should not be perceived as a weakness by the physician.

UNIQUE APPROACHES TO FIGHTING PHYSICIAN BURNOUT

As described previously, over 80 factors have been identified as risk factors for physician burnout. Isolating and targeting primary factors is difficult for organizations that often do not have the interest, time, or resources to invest. Therefore, individual work units or physicians should actively evaluate their own work environment to prevent fatigue and burnout. One approach is for an individual or group to actively investigate risks and possible interventions by understanding the motivational theory of Maslow's hierarchy of needs. This model utilizes a 5-tier pyramidal structure. The lower two tiers include basic needs such as food, water, and safety. Once these needs are met, a person can climb to tiers 3 and 4, which describe psychological needs such as relationships and accomplishments. The last tier includes self-fulfillment needs. In this tiered model one cannot skip levels if needs at a lower level are unmet.[52] In 2019, an adapted model called the Health Professional Wellness Hierarchy was created and published to directly target the needs of the physician and to avert burnout. This model assumes that health professionals are motivated by a desire to deliver high-quality care to their patients but under the premise that their basic needs and personal enjoyment are met (**Fig. 1**).[24] This brilliant model forces physicians to actively gain insight into their own workplace stressors. This model has been further adapted specifically to address resident wellness needs and stress home relationships, mentorship, and additional educational opportunities.[53]

Another easy approach is for physicians to recognize that work-induced fatigue will be experienced during their career and that stressors will change over time. Active investigation utilizing targeted themed questions should give physicians self-awareness and insight into immediate threats for their wellbeing. Global questions can be utilized to uncover categories of stress (**Box 1**). Interventions for immediate threats should be actionable and measurable and reflect the current work unit stressor (**Box 2**). Individual stressors and their interventions should be assessed on an ongoing basis and should be modified if success is not accomplished.

THE COVID-19 PANDEMIC: A NEW CHALLENGE FOR PHYSICIAN BURNOUT

The COVID-19 pandemic caused by severe acute respiratory syndrome coronavirus 2 originated in Wuhan, China, and was first recognized by the World Health Organization in December 2019. By December 31st of 2020, more than 82 million people had contracted the virus and over 1.8 million people worldwide had died from complications of the virus.[54] Healthcare workers have been at the front line of the pandemic with COVID-related hospitalizations skyrocketing. Procedural-related specialties saw an unprecedented downturn in their practice with elective procedures being universally halted for months.

This pandemic has led to additional stresses placed on already fatigued physicians, with frontline physicians in the fields of critical care and emergency medicine being hit especially hard. An email survey of emergency medicine physicians found the median burnout and exhaustion measure increased from prepandemic levels by 1.8 points (scale of 1–7). Over 90% stated they had a change in behavior toward friends and family. The most common reasons for stress were concern for lack of availability of

Title	Level	Key factors at level

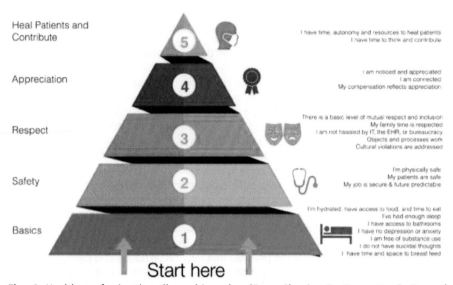

Heal Patients and Contribute — 5 — I have time, autonomy and resources to heal patients / I have time to think and contribute

Appreciation — 4 — I am noticed and appreciated / I am connected / My compensation reflects appreciation

Respect — 3 — There is a basic level of mutual respect and inclusion / My family time is respected / I am not hassled by IT, the EHR, or bureaucracy / Objects and processes work / Cultural violations are addressed

Safety — 2 — I'm physically safe / My patients are safe / My job is secure & future predictable

Basics — 1 — I'm hydrated, have access to food, and time to eat / I've had enough sleep / I have access to bathrooms / I have no depression or anxiety / I am free of substance use / I do not have suicidal thoughts / I have time and space to breast feed

Start here

Fig. 1. Health professional wellness hierarchy. (*From* Shapiro D, Duquette C. Beyond Burnout: A Physician Wellness Hierarchy Designed to Prioritize I interventions at the Systems Level. Am J Med 2019;132:556–563; with permission.)

personal protective equipment, lack of rapid testing, and leave for taking care of family and self.[55] Women and unmarried trainees have suffered the most negative consequences, with the highest levels of burnout.[56] Childcare, unpaid domestic labor, and adjustments in work are strong factors in this gender disparity.[57,58] Exposure to COVID-19 patients also increased anxiety and stress. A survey of trainees revealed that trainees exposed to patients with COVID-19 experienced significantly higher stress and burnout than trainees with no exposure.[59]

Job security and income have also been major stresses on physicians who are already on the front lines of care for COVID-19 patients. A survey by Merritt Hawkins, a physician recruitment firm, found that over 20% of physician were either furloughed

---

Box 1
Physician fatigue questionnaire

- Do you feel burdened by the electronic medical record or clerical/nonphysician-related tasks?
- Do you feel that the workflow at work is inefficient or stressful?
- Do you feel that your direct leader does not support your job- or work-related issues?
- Do you believe your work hour requirements are stressful or that you spend too much time doing work that is not meaningful to you?
- Are you overwhelmed by potential medical errors or possible litigation?
- Are you worried that you are not competent in procedures or in your area of expertise?

Box 2
Physician fatigue intervention algorithm

Administrative burdens (EMR, required training modules, work emails)
- Dedicated time to address administrative burdens
- Utilization of medical scribes
- Peer mentors or trainers to teach EMR efficiency (both physician and peer mentor need dedicated time for this)

Workflow (inefficiency and stress related directly to patient care)
- Cross-train staff
- Ensure adequate training and number of staff
- Empower and insist staff take on nonphysician clerical work (forms, EMR data entry, faxing, authorizations)
- Restructure work units to match staff with physicians
- Restructure patient care time intervals
- Restructure preoperative care team duties to engender teamwork and efficiency
- Engage leadership for needed resources (parking, PPE, childcare, sleeping)

Ineffective leadership
- Regular rotation of leadership
- 360 evaluations of leaders
- Formal coaching for the leader
- Regularly scheduled team meetings with all personnel levels

Work hours/monotony
- Flexible work hours
- 4-day work week
- Protected time
- Altered schedule/shifts for inpatient work
- Dedicated time for work deemed "meaningful'
- Reassessment of compensation model with leadership

Fear of medical errors, litigation, procedural competence
- Peer groups
- Mentorship
- Internal workshops
- Subsidized continuing education courses
- Dedicated physician space/lounge

---

or received pay cuts during the pandemic. Overall, 14% of physicians stated they wanted to leave their practice, while another 6% wanted to leave medicine entirely.[59]

COMBATING BURNOUT DURING THE COVID PANDEMIC

Unique institutional initiatives during COVID-19 are paramount to combating physician burnout.[60] A listening study evaluating concerns of healthcare professionals during COVID found that healthcare professionals appreciated leaders that were visible, understood ongoing challenges, supported staff by asking what they need, and expressed gratitude. Recognizing and listening to physician expertise and making physicians part of the decision-making process regarding testing, procedural protocols, and needed equipment have been essential during this crisis. Providing adequate personal protective equipment and ensuring rapid testing for COVID exposures should also be a top priority. Supporting physicians on the front line with adequate housing, food, water, and transportation needs can prevent burnout. Assisting with childcare needs, flexible work hours, emotional support, direct counseling, and webinars should also be considered.[61]

SUMMARY

Physician fatigue, also known as burnout, is a highly prevalent but often underrecognized result of workplace stressors. The consequences of burnout can include poor work–life integration, isolation, depression, and suicide. As a result, an organization may experience high physician turnover, patient safety issues, malpractice suits, and financial losses. Physicians should be encouraged to play a role in their wellness by taking mental time away from work, pursuing hobbies, attending wellness programs, and by ensuring dedicated quality time with family. Ultimately, it is an organization that must acknowledge physician burnout, identify risk factors, and invest in targeted interventions to prevent this immense threat to their stability.

CLINICS CARE POINTS

- Physician fatigue, also known as burnout, is a direct result of workplace stressors.
- Physician burnout is often underrecognized by both the physician and his/her organization.
- Main risk factors for burnout include administrative hassles, work-flow inefficiencies, work hour burdens, and ineffective leadership.
- Physician burnout can lead to depression, suicide, and poor work–life integration.
- Self-directed interventions such as wellness programs may be helpful but alone may not be enough to prevent burnout.
- Organizations must acknowledge physician burnout as a threat to their financial stability requiring ongoing focused workplace interventions.

DISCLOSURE

The author has nothing to disclose.

REFERENCES

1. Freudenberger HJ. The staff burn-out syndrome in alternative institutions. Psychotherapy 1975;12(1):73–82.
2. Maslach C, Jackson SE. The measurement of experienced burnout. J Occup Behav 1981;2:99–113.
3. Dyrbye LN, Satele D. Utility of a brief screening tool to identify physicians in distress. J Gen Intern Med 2012;28(3):421–7.
4. ICD-11 for Mortality and Morbidity Statistics (Version: 09/2020). Available at: https://icd.who.int/browse11/l-m/en#/http%3a%2f%2fid.who.int%2ficd%2fentity%2f129180281. Accessed December 10, 2020.
5. Brazeau CM, Shanafelt. Distress among matriculating medical students relative to the general population. Acad Med 2019;89:1520–5.
6. Dyrbye L, West CP. Burnout among US medical students, residents, and early career physicians relative to the general US population. Acad Med 2014;89(3):443–51.
7. DeCross AJ. How to approach burnout among Gastroenterology fellows. Gastroenterology 2020;158:32–5.
8. Rotenstein LS, Torre M. Prevalence of burnout among physicians: A systematic review. JAMA 2018;320(11):1131–50.
9. Shanafelt TD, Boone S. Archives of Internal Medicine. Burnout and Satisfaction with work-life balance among US physicians relative to the general US population. Arch Intern Med 2012;172(18):1377–85.

10. Peckham C. Physician Burnout: It Just Keeps Getting Worse. Physician Lifestyle Report. 2015. Available at: https://www.medscape.com/features. Accessed November 15, 2020.

11. Barnes EL, Ketwaroo GA. Scope of burnout among young gastroenterologists and practical solutions from gastroenterology and other disciplines. Dig Dis Sci 2019;64:302–6.

12. Keswani RN, Keefer RN. Burnout in gastroenterologists and How to Prevent it. Gastroenterology 2014;147:11–4.

13. Campbell DA, Sonnad SS. Burnout among American Surgeons. Surgery 2001; 130(4):696–705.

14. Keswani RN, Taft TH. Increased levels of stress and burnout are related to decreased physician experience and to interventional gastroenterology career choice: findings from a US survey of endoscopists. Am Coll Gastroenterol 2011;106:1734–40.

15. Schernhammer ES, Colditz GA. Suicide rates among physicians: A quantitative and gender assessment (meta-analysis). Am J Psychiatry 2004;161:2295–302.

16. Schernhammer ES. Taking their own lives: the high rate of physician suicide. N Engl J Med 2005;352(24):2473–6.

17. Hawton K, Malmberg A. Suicide in doctors. A psychological autopsy studies. J Psychosom Res 2004;57:1–4.

18. Fink-Miller EL, Nestler LM. Suicide in physicians and veterinarians: risk factors and theories. Curr Opin Psychol 2018;22:23–6.

19. Keeton K, Fenner DE. Predictors of physician career satisfaction, work–life balance, and burnout. Obstet Gyn 2007;109(4):949–55.

20. Shanafelt TD, Hasan O. Changes in burnout and satisfaction with work-life balance in physicians and the general US working population between 2011 and 2014. Mayo Clin Proc 2015;12:1600–13.

21. Shanafelt TD, Boone SL. The medical marriage: a national survey of the spouses/partners of US physicians. Mayo Clinic Proc 2013;88(3):216–25.

22. Ly D, Seabury S. Divorce among physicians and other healthcare professionals in the United States: analysis of census survey data. BMJ 2015;350:h706.

23. Shanafelt T, Hasan O. Parental satisfaction of US physicians: associated factors and comparison with the general US working population. Bmc Med Education 2016;16:228.

24. Shapiro D, Duquette C. Beyond burnout: a physician wellness hierarchy designed to prioritize i interventions at the systems level. Am J Med 2019;132: 556–63.

25. Arndt BG, Beasley JW. Tethered to the EHR: primary care physician workload assessment using EHR event log data and time-motion observations. Ann Fam Med 2017;15:419–26.

26. Melnick ER, Dyrbye LN. The association between perceived electronic health record usability and professional burnout among US physicians. Mayo Clinic Proc 2020;95(3):476–87.

27. Jacobs CM. Ineffective-leader induced occupational stress. SAGE Open 2019;1–15.

28. Barling J. If only my leader would just do something! Passive leadership undermines employee well-being through role stressors and psychological resource depletion. Stress and Health 2016;33(3):211–22.

29. Shanafelt TD, Gorringe J. Impact of organizational leadership on physician burnout and satisfaction. Mayo Clin Proc 2015;90(4):432–40.

30. Gerstenberger PD, Plumeri PA. Malpractice claims in gastrointestinal endoscopy: analysis of insurance industry data base. Gastrointest Endosc 1993;39(2):132–8.

31. Hamidi MS, Bohman B. Estimating institutional physician turnover attributable to self-reported burnout and associated financial burden: a case study. BMC Health Serv Res 2018;18:851.

32. Hans S, Shanafelt T. Estimating the attributable cost of physician burnout in the United States. Ann Intern Med 2019;170:784–90.

33. Panagiotti M, Geraghty K. Association between physician burnout and patient safety, professionalism, and patient satisfaction. A systematic review and meta-analysis. JAMA Intern Med 2018;178(10):1317–30.

34. Anagnostopoulos F, Liolios E. Physician burnout and patient satisfaction with consultation in primary health care settings: evidence of relationships from a one-with-many design. J Clin Psychol Med Settings 2012;19(4):401–10.

35. Shanafelt TD, Kaups KL. An interactive individualized intervention to promote behavioral change to increase personal well-being in US surgeons. Ann Surg 2014;259(1):82–8.

36. Leiter MP, Maslach C. Latent burnout profiles: A new approach to understanding the burnout experience. Burnout Res 2016;3(4):89–100.

37. West CP, Dyrbye LN. Single item measures of emotional exhaustion and depersonalization are useful for assessing burnout in medical professionals. J Gen Intern Med 2009;24:1318–21.

38. Dzau VJ, Kirch DG. To care is human: Collectively confronting the clinician-burnout crisis. N Engl J Med 2018;378(4):312–4.

39. Noseworthy J, Madara J. Physician burnout is a public health crisis: A message to our fellow health care CEOs. Health Affairs Blog. 2017. Available at. https://www.healthaffairs.org/do/10.1377/hblog20170328.059397/full/. Accessed December 20, 2020.

40. Shanafelt TD, Noseworthy JN. Executive leadership and physician well-being: Nine organizational strategies to promote engagement and reduce burnout. Mayo Clin Proc 2017;92(1):129–46.

41. Panagioti M, Panagopoulou E. Controlled Interventions to reduce burnout in physicians. A systematic review and meta-analysis. JAMA Int Med 2017;177(2):95–205.

42. Linzer M, Poplau S. A cluster randomized trial of interventions to improve work conditions and clinician burnout in primary care, results from the Healthy Workplace (HWP) study. J Gen Intern Med 2015;30(8):1105–11.

43. Yang AD, Chung JW. Differences in resident perceptions by postgraduate year of duty hour policies: an analysis from the flexibility in duty hour requirements for surgical trainees (FIRST) trial. J Am Coll Surg 2017;224:103–12.

44. Shanafelt TD, West CP. Career fit and burnout among academic faculty. Arch Intern Med 2009;169:990–5.

45. Zhou H, Sheng X. Ethical leadership as the reliever of frontline service employees' emotional exhaustion: A moderated mediation. Int J Environ Res Public Health 2020;17:976.

46. Dyrbye LN, Shanafelt TD. Effect of professional coaching intervention on the well-being and distress of physicians. A pilot randomized clinical trial. JAMA Intern Med 2019;1406–11.

47. Taft TH, Keefer L. Friends, alcohol, and a higher power: an analysis of adaptive and maladaptive coping strategies among gastroenterologists. J Clin Gastroenterol 2011;45(8):76–81.

48. West CP, Dyrbye LN. Intervention to promote physician well-being, job satisfaction and professionalism. A randomized clinical trial. JAMA 2014;174(4):527–33.
49. Lacy BE, Chan JL. Physician burnout. The hidden health crisis. Clin Gastroenterol Hepatol 2018;16:311–7.
50. Shanafelt TD, Oreskovich MR. Avoiding burnout: the personal health habits and wellness practices of US Surgeons. Ann Surg 2012;255(4):625–33.
51. Krasner MS, Epstein RM. Association of an educational program in mindful communication with burnout, empathy, and attitudes among primary care physicians. JAMA 2009;302(12):1284–93.
52. Maslow AH. A theory of human motivation. Psychol Rev 1943;50(4):370–96.
53. Hale AJ, Ricotta DN. Adapting Maslow's hierarchy of needs as a framework for resident wellness. Teach Learn Med 2019;31:109–18.
54. Accessed from website Johns Hopkins Coronavirus Resource Center (jhu.edu) on Dec 31, 2020.
55. Rodriquez RM, Medak AJ. Academic emergency medicine physicians' anxiety levels, stressors, and potential stress mitigation measures during the acceleration phase of the COVID-19 pandemic. Acad Emerg Med 2020;27(8):700–7.
56. Kannampallil TG, Goss CW. Exposure to COVID-19 patients increases physician trainee stress and burnout. 2020. Available at online at PLOS ONE. https://doi.org/10.1371/journal.pone.0237301. Accessed December 20, 2020.
57. Easing the COVID-19 burden on working parents'. BCG Global. 2020. Available at. https://www.bcg.com/publications/2020/helping-working-parents-ease-the-burden-of-covid-19. Accessed December 01, 2020.
58. Brubaker L. Women Physicians and the COVID Pandemic. JAMA 2020;324(9):835–6.
59. Rapier G. One in 5 doctors has been furloughed or taken a pay cut as the coronavirus pandemic hits hospitals. Some say they're considering New Jobs. Business Insider. 2020. Available at: https://www.businessinsider.in/science/health/news. Accessed December 20, 2020.
60. Amanullah S, Shankar RR. The impact of COVID-19 on physician burnout globally: a review. Healthcare 2020;421:8.
61. Shanafelt TD, Ripp J. Understanding and addressing sources of anxiety among health care professionals during the COVID-19 pandemic. JAMA 2020;323(21):2133–4.

Ergonomics of Endoscopy

Anna M. Lipowska, MD[a],*, Amandeep K. Shergill, MD, MS[b]

KEYWORDS

- Ergonomics • Musculoskeletal injury • Endoscopy unit • Injury prevention
- Personal protective equipment • Occupational safety

KEY POINTS

- Incorporation of ergonomic principles into the endoscopy environment is essential and benefits endoscopists, endoscopy unit personnel, and patients.
- Thoughtful planning of procedure schedules creates time for microbreaks and a preprocedural ergonomic time-out.
- Ergonomic training programs ideally incorporate the entire endoscopy staff, including trainees, practicing endoscopists, nurses, and technicians.
- Optimal procedure room design encompasses adaptable equipment and reduction of workplace hazards.

INTRODUCTION

The endoscopy environment is a complex setting where numerous patients receive care, endoscopy personnel balance a multifaceted work flow, and endoscopists perform rigorous physically demanding tasks. Incorporation of ergonomic principles into the endoscopy environment is essential. Ergonomics is the science of designing a job to fit the individual, instead of forcing an individual to fit a job. This article presents ergonomically focused goals for the endoscopy operations team.

Thoughtful design of the entire endoscopy unit environment uses a user-centered approach that allows for flexibility, privacy, comfort, and safety. Ergonomically minded scheduling and endoscopic ergonomics training programs can benefit all team members. Furthermore, investing in ancillary tools and new technologies may help facilitate the efficient and safe performance of endoscopy. Benefits of ergonomics reach beyond a reduction of musculoskeletal injury (MSI) and include increased productivity, fewer lost work days, decreased burnout, and improved job satisfaction and well-being.

[a] Division of Gastroenterology and Hepatology, University of Illinois at Chicago, 840 South Wood Street, CSB Suite 741 (MC 716), Chicago, IL 60612, USA; [b] Division of Gastroenterology and Hepatology, San Francisco Veterans Affairs Medical Center and University of California, 4150 Clement Street, VA 111B/ GI Section, San Francisco, CA 94121, USA
* Corresponding author.
E-mail address: lipowska@uic.edu

Gastrointest Endoscopy Clin N Am 31 (2021) 655–669
https://doi.org/10.1016/j.giec.2021.05.003
1052-5157/21/© 2021 Elsevier Inc. All rights reserved.

giendo.theclinics.com

INJURY RISKS AMONG ENDOSCOPISTS AND MECHANISMS OF INJURY

A high prevalence of occupational MSI is well established among gastroenterologists. Endoscopy requires performance of repetitive motions, prolonged awkward postures, and sustained high pinch force. Resulting recurring microtrauma to the body can lead to overuse injuries.[1] Nonneutral postures decrease a muscle's ability to generate maximal force and thus result in lower tissue tolerances. Repetitive, high-force loading, especially in nonneutral postures, can overcome the internal tissue tolerances of the muscles, tendons, ligaments, fascia, bursa, and nerves and lead to tissue inflammation and remodeling.[2] If the tissue is not deloaded and given adequate time for proper healing, this can result in inadequate cellular and matrix repair, scarring, and loss of tissue strength and integrity.[3] A systematic review revealed that 39% to 89% of surveyed gastrointestinal endoscopists reported endoscopy-related MSI.[4] In the European population, a large study demonstrated a 69.6% prevalence of endoscopy-related MSI, with the neck being most frequently affected.[5] Notably, an independent association was observed between female gender and MSI and severe pain.

A biomechanical analysis of distal upper extremity exposures during colonoscopy demonstrated high-risk exposures that provide a rationale for the development of endoscopy-related pain in the thumbs, hands, and elbows as well as for carpal tunnel syndrome.[6] In this study, female endoscopists tended to apply a higher right pinch force with greater right forearm muscle activity throughout the colonoscopy procedure than male endoscopists. Females, who tend to have smaller hands, may be unable to reach the right/left dial controls with their left thumb as easily as males and may instead relay on manipulation of the insertion tube by the right distal upper extremity. Thus, hand dimensions likely play a significant role in the interaction of the left hand with the control section of the endoscope and overall scope handling and should be considered as part of a user-centered design approach. Gastroenterology trainees are not exempt from injury in spite of shorter duration in practice. A survey study of this group noted that 20% of fellows experience MSI, with female gender a risk factor for injury.[7]

ERGONOMIC EDUCATION

The importance of ergonomic education and training is widely recognized.[8,9] While a deeper analysis of optimal scope handling is beyond the scope of this publication, both trainees as well as practicing gastroenterologists benefit from ergonomic guidance to optimize their posture and performance. In the trainee population, an ergonomic training curriculum was associated with diminished endoscopy-related MSI risk as assessed by ergonomic risk-assessment tools.[10] The growing number of long and technically complex procedures within gastroenterology further highlights the need for a strong ergonomic foundation.[11,12] Combining optimization of the endoscopy suite environment with instruction on advantageous endoscopic techniques decreases the risk of potential overuse injuries.[13]

Team-wide educational initiatives can also improve ergonomic awareness. Training programs incorporating informational videos, interactive sessions on optimal room setup, and instructive reading materials have demonstrated benefit in improving endoscopic ergonomic knowledge.[14] Importantly, inclusion of the entire team allows them to become part of the solution.

Multiple resources are available to help endoscopy units build a strong ergonomic foundation and include

- The ASGE video "Ergonomic Essentials for your Practice"[15]

- The VideoGIE series on endoscopy ergonomics by Cheng and colleagues[16–18] (https://www.videogie.org/article/S2468-4481(17)30063-2/fulltext) (https://www.videogie.org/article/S2468-4481(17)30064-4/fulltext) (https://www.videogie.org/article/S2468-4481(17)30065-6/fulltext)
- Hospital-based ergonomics programs

DESIGN OF THE PATIENT CARE ENVIRONMENT

Thoughtful design of the endoscopy center's patient care environment that incorporates basic ergonomic principles can optimize efficiency, patient care team satisfaction, and safety (**Fig. 1**). The patient care space includes three main sections: preprocedure area, procedure area, and postprocedure area (**Table 1**). The goal is

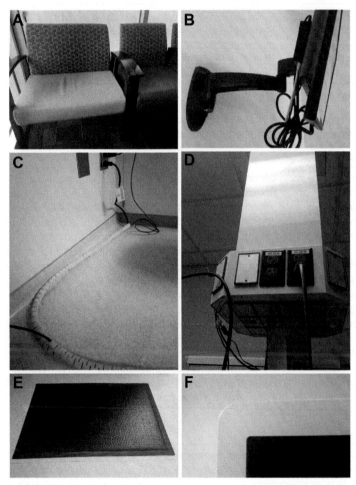

Fig. 1. Thoughtful design elements of the endoscopy center incorporating ergonomic principles. (*A*) Spacious seating accommodates all patients. (*B*) Bundling cords creates an uncluttered environment. (*C*) Avoiding exposed wires and tubing helps prevent tripping. (*D*) Roof mounting electrical outlets and cords keeps them off the floor. (*E*) Cushioned floor mat with down sloping edges decreases standing fatigue. (*F*) Monitor with rounded edges.

Table 1
Patient care area design suggestions

Patient Care Areas		
Preprocedure Area	**Procedure Area**	**Postprocedure Area**
Waiting Room	*Procedure Room Design*	*Recovery Area*
Spacious doorways and seating	Adaptable monitor position vertically and horizontally	Equipment available and uncluttered
Warm lighting and colors	Adjustable bed height	Proximal to nurses' station
Gentle music	Close fluoroscopy and endoscopy monitors	Emergency cart access
Nature components	Slip-resistant flooring	Accessible restrooms
Privacy and space	Bundled cords and tubing	Staff escort
Preparation Area	*Procedure Room Accessories*	
Uncluttered and clean	Floor cushion support	
Barriers between patient beds	Accessible pedal positioning	
Accessible restrooms	Raised surface/stool	
Proximal to nurses' station	Personal accessories	

© 2021 Anna Lipowska

to achieve organized flow of the patient and staff from one area to the next, with minimal crossover points and maximal productivity.

Preprocedure Area

The preprocedure zone encompasses the reception desk, waiting room, and the patient preparation area. Spacious doorways and seating will accommodate wheelchairs, individuals with disabilities, the elderly, and patients of all body habitus. Welcoming interior design features including warm lighting and paint colors may help diminish preprocedure anxiety.[19] The existence of positive distractions such as videos of travel and nature programs as well as gentle music can decrease overstimulation and perceived waiting time.[20] Nature components including greenery, windows, fish tanks, and water features can also provide a sense of well-being. Importantly, sufficient privacy and space is critical.

In the patient preparation area, intake is performed, and patients are readied for their procedures. As this is a vulnerable zone, it is important to maintain patient confidentiality and privacy with adequate barriers between patient beds. Mounting equipment on the wall, such as adjustable computers and patient monitors, and bundling wires can contribute to a clean and uncluttered environment while minimizing risk of falls.[21] Bathrooms with handicap and bariatric accessibility should be located nearby. Close proximity to the nurses' station allows patients to reach their care team if in need and improves communication.

Procedure Area

Ergonomic design of the procedure room is crucial as this is where endoscopists spend the majority of their time and are at most risk of work-related MSI. Adjustability is key to allow endoscopists to maintain neutral body postures and sustain performance during potentially long and complex procedures.[13] The increasing number of women entering the field of gastroenterology highlights the importance of adaptability to a wide range of statures. Optimal room design uses anthropometric data to accommodate the 5th percentile female to the 95th percentile male.[22]

Room setup

An ergonomic stance during endoscopy involves neutral neck and back position without hyperextension or flexion, even weight distribution between both legs, and avoidance of knee hyperextension. Persistent lumbar flexion can lead to an increased lumbar load and risk of spinal compression.[23] For the upper extremities, it has been shown that forearm orientation affects wrist joint biomechanics.[24]

The monitor should be located directly in front of the endoscopist to minimize neck torsion. To maintain vertical neutral neck position, the center of the screen should fall at 15 to 25° below eye level and accommodate the resting eye angle.[1] Within the anthropometric range, this translates to monitor adjustability between 93 and 162 cm from the floor. Keeping the monitor too close or too far can contribute to eye strain. Depending on monitor quality and specifications, favorable distance between the monitor and the proceduralists is estimated between 52 and 182 cm. The monitors themselves should possess rounded edges to lessen harm in case of accidental physical contact.

When holding the endoscope, the elbows should bend near a 90° angle with the insertion tube located at or 10 cm below elbow height.[1] To accommodate neutral body position for a variety of body builds, the examination table should be height adjustable between 85 and 120 cm from the floor to minimize forward flexion or shoulder abduction.

Flooring

The floor of the endoscopy suite can be the source of accidental occupational injuries.[21] Exposed wires, cords, and tubing may lead the endoscopy personnel to trip and fall. It is strongly recommended that cords be bundled together and covered when possible. Ceiling-mounted plugs decrease the number of floor-bound cords. Altering flooring to have a slip-resistant quality can also prevent workplace injuries.[25]

Thoughtful use of floor accessories can promote ergonomic standards. Floor pedals for cautery and water jets should be easily accessible and within reach without straining. Many endoscopic procedures require prolonged standing. Cushion support such as mats with down sloping edges serve to reduce back strain and leg discomfort.[26] Alternating posture by placing one's foot onto a stool or raised surface can minimize static loads. Personal accessories such as wearing cushioned insoles and compression stockings encourage postural changes and may increase circulation during a long procedure.[27,28]

Postprocedure Area

Recovery and ultimately discharge after endoscopy occurs in the postprocedure area. Ergonomic workstation design is critical to ensure staff are able to monitor patients safely and complete necessary paperwork efficiently. On arrival, most patients are sedated, thus unobstructed visibility of patients from the nurses' station is vital to maximize safety. In the event of an emergency, a crash cart should be maintained close by without blocking passages and entryways. All recovery equipment, while within reach, should be organized in an orderly and uncluttered fashion. Patients may need to use bathroom facilities after procedures. Proximity of the lavatory and staff availability to escort patients and decrease fall risk are important considerations.

SCHEDULING

In addition to the physical endoscopy unit design, the endoscopy schedule and workflow are important considerations (**Box 1**). Studies have demonstrated that increased procedure volume, hours per week performing procedures, and cumulative time in

---

Box 1
Endoscopy culture practices with a focus on an ergonomically favored schedule and work flow

Ergonomic scheduling and workflow considerations
- Ergonomic time-out
- Microbreaks
- Schedule design
- Importance of physical fitness
- Stretching exercises

---

practice are associated with increased risk of procedural occupational injury.[4,5,11] Furthermore, MSI have been found to impact productivity leading practicing gastroenterologists to decrease procedural volume or miss days of work.[4,5]

There is no defined maximum number of procedures that can be performed safely because of great variance in individual and practice characteristics. Endoscopists are advised to pay attention to any symptoms and limit exertion if experiencing pain that may be related to MSI. Half instead of full endoscopy procedure days may be considered, and spacing out endoscopy sessions in the week permits additional recovery time. Importantly, endoscopists should not be experiencing pain from a prior endoscopy session when starting another endoscopy session. Optimal scheduling within a day of endoscopy allows for adequate breaks between cases and supports a culture where rest is normalized.[29,30] Even microbreaks lasting 1 to 2 minutes have been shown to improve performance and reduce pain.[31] Unfortunately, most endoscopists do not take regular breaks, with one survey reporting that only 10% of respondents scheduled regular breaks.[11]

Integration of an ergonomic time-out into the procedure work flow ensures optimization of room setup before the procedure begins.[32] Adding just a few seconds to run through the Ergonomic Checklist can verify optimal equipment and room setup (**Box 2**). Stretching and exercise can be incorporated in between procedures and after completion of the day's cases. While data are limited on the benefits of stretching on endoscopy-related injury, advantages of stretching leading to injury prevention are established in other physically demanding roles such as athletics. Stretching can be used for injury prevention and to maintain flexibility and strength. Educational materials on postprocedural exercises that have been adapted to the endoscopy unit are available.[15,33]

ADVANCED ENDOSCOPY

Advanced endoscopy comes with its own unique challenges and specialized equipment, and several survey-based studies report a high prevalence of injuries in

---

Box 2
Ergonomic checklist

Ergonomic checklist
- Monitor placed directly in front
- Monitor 15 to 25° below eye level
- Raised procedure bed bringing endoscope to 10 cm below elbow height
- Floor cushion in place
- Floor pedal in front of body
- Back, upper and lower extremities in neutral position
- 2-piece lead apron preferred (if using)
- Cords and wires contained on floor
- Implementation of microbreaks and stretching

Courtesy of Anna Lipowska, MD, Chicago, IL.

---

advanced endoscopists.[34,35] Given advanced endoscopists' high rates of musculo-skeletal disorders, implementation of ergonomically focused preventative strategies is important to minimize injury.[36]

Advanced procedure rooms should be large enough to accommodate the utilization of the c-arm fluoroscope and the larger number of ancillary staff required to perform complex procedures, including the anesthesiology team. For procedures using fluoroscopy, the endoscopy team members must wear a protective lead apron, which places additional loads on the trunk muscles and intravertebral discs.[37] These are available in a variety of profiles including one-piece, two-piece, and pregnancy aprons. Two-piece lead aprons have been found to produce less discomfort by redistributing a portion of the weight across the hips from the upper body.[38] Fluoroscopy often requires the use of two monitors or inputs, necessitating the endoscopist to turn their necks throughout the study. Placement of the endoscopy and fluoroscopy monitors close together has been found to prevent neck torsion and decrease eye strain and total fluoroscopy time.[36,39]

INVESTMENT IN TECHNOLOGY

There is a growing interest in innovative strategies to reduce risk of injury related to endoscope design. Development and production of the endoscope and accessory tools should incorporate ergonomic principles. The current endoscope design is one-size-fits all and does not accommodate the range of hand strengths and sizes of the breadth of female and male endoscopists. The growth of therapeutic endoscopy has driven endoscope evolution, and the majority of the changes to the endoscope have focused on image quality, image processing, and the insertion tube. The control section has not changed significantly since the 1980s.[40] Studies in the field of surgery have examined laparoscopic tool performance and design from an ergonomic perspective.[41,42] Future endoscope redesign should incorporate human factors and explore instrument adaptability to various hand dimensions. In addition, each endoscopy unit should have a rigorous endoscope maintenance program to preserve optimal instrument function and responsiveness for the safety of the proceduralist and the patient.

Several accessory devices have been developed to support the endoscope and endoscopic technique. Endoscope support stands aim to reduce the static load of the endoscope's control section. The use of an antigravity support arm during simulated colonoscopy demonstrated a reduction in left extensor loads.[6] Angulation assist dials aim to bring controls within a more comfortable reach for smaller hand sizes, although to date, there is a lack of a clear demonstrated intraprocedural benefit in the literature. While more data are needed to verify the advantages of these ancillary devices before widespread use, these tools may assist endoscopists who are experiencing difficulty holding or manipulating the control section.

Adjustable monitors and beds are required to ensure endoscopists can attain a neutral posture of the neck, back, and shoulders. All endoscopy units should invest in adjustable monitor arms, stands, or ceiling booms that allow the room setup to be optimized for the range of endoscopist heights.

BEYOND THE ENDOSCOPIST: ERGONOMICS FOR THE ENDOSCOPY TEAM

The importance of ergonomics transcends beyond the endoscopist. Nurses and gastroenterology technicians are part of the endoscopy team and are influenced by ergonomic practices. Inclusion of every member of the team in ergonomic initiatives fosters a culture of safety and promotes injury prevention.

Injury Risks Among Endoscopy Nurses

Similar to endoscopists, endoscopy nurses face hazards in the workplace including the potential for MSI. While nurses across many departments report physical occupational demands, the endoscopy environment brings unique challenges. Endoscopy staff facilitate fast patient turnover, transport patients and perform repetitive work when documenting on computers, sedating and monitoring patients, and assisting with tools during endoscopy procedures. Nurses and technicians may perform ancillary maneuvers such as changing patient position or applying abdominal compression to facilitate cecal intubation.

Examination of upper extremity injuries among endoscopy nurses demonstrate a high prevalence of upper extremity, neck and back complaints, requiring analgesic use and medical treatment and resulting in work absences.[43–46] Full-time work was positively associated with disability.[44] Factoring in turnaround time to staff scheduling was linked to lower upper extremity disability scores.[45] In one study, a secondary analysis suggested a range of interventions to mitigate risk including task rotation, evaluation of staffing levels, organization support, and device usability, among others.[46] The availability of ergonomic and physiotherapy assessments as well as disposable turning and lifting devices was found to be associated with lower neck and back disability scores.[47]

Patient Handling

It is well established that repetitive patient handling and lifting can increase the risk of musculoskeletal disorders.[48] During endoscopy, patients frequently require repositioning and are limited in their ability to do so independently because of the effects of sedation. The entire endoscopy team may be involved in moving patients during the procedure with limited visibility in dim lighting. To start, individuals should avoid lifting beyond their capabilities. While there are no strict weight limits for lifting tasks, the National Institute for Occupational Safety and Health advises caution beyond a 35-lbs load.[49] For individuals, proper lift techniques include the use of hips and knees, a wide base, and minimizing forward flexion to reduce back strain. The use of lifting equipment and slide sheets for patient transfer should be encouraged. Rotating responsibilities and adequate team support may also reduce exposures and risk (**Box 3**).

Abdominal Compression

During endoscopy, application of abdominal compression by nurses or technicians is frequently used to facilitate cecal intubation in the case of looping during colonoscopy. A study of endoscopy nurses in the United States demonstrated that on average, abdominal pressure is applied for 6.3 minutes per colonoscopy case.[45] While no standardized approach currently exists, suggested strategies to minimize risk of injury include applying specific instead of general pressure, keeping the wrist in neutral position by using the forearm, combining pressure application with other tactics such as gentle suction and stiffening of the insertion tube and repositioning the patient to improve access[50,51] (**Box 4**).

The challenges of transabdominal compression delivery have led to the development of assistive devices to substitute manual pressure application. Multiple randomized controlled trials examining abdominal compression devices reported potential benefits including decreased cecal intubation time.[52,53] A blinded randomized controlled trial of abdominal compression assistive devices compared a sham device to the ColoWrap binder.[54] This study found that in patients undergoing elective colonoscopy, application of the device did not improve cecal intubation time or affect the

---

Box 3
Patient handling tips for lifting and transferring patients

Patient lifting and transfer considerations
- Use of slide sheets, body lifts, slings
- Safe lift technique
- Avoidance of awkward postures
- Refraining from twisting while lifting
- Short duration of lifting
- Rotating responsibilities
- Adequate team and management support

---

frequency of ancillary maneuvers. A subgroup analysis suggested a possible benefit in patients with a body mass index between 30 and 40 kg/m^2. While abdominal binders are a promising technology that may lead to benefits in a select population, more data are needed to support its routine use for ergonomic benefit.

The Society for Gastrointestinal Nursing recently published a position statement on ergonomics in the gastroenterology setting.[55] To promote a culture of safety, endoscopy operations management is encouraged to develop and execute safe patient handling policies and focus on quality improvement and wellness. Education on basic ergonomic principles should be cultivated and made available to all staff. This team approach allows everyone to buy into safety practices and optimizes endoscopy suite function. Importantly, all staff should be aware of the potential for work-related injury and pay attention to any symptoms that may indicate the development of MSI.

COVID-19 AND PERSONAL PROTECTIVE EQUIPMENT (PPE) IN ENDOSCOPY

SARS-CoV-2, the virus that causes COVID-19, is spread via droplets carrying infectious viral particles. Routes of infection include contact transmission, droplet transmission, and airborne transmission.[56] Endoscopy is an aerosol-generating procedure, and the GI tract is a potential reservoir of infection, with persistent positive stool test results even after nasal polymerase chain reaction has turned negative.[57,58] To minimize risk of spread during endoscopy, additional infection control practices have been recommended which include the use of the enhanced PPE and additional respiratory protection during endoscopy to minimize risk of airborne spread.

Updated PPE recommendations for performing endoscopy during the COVID pandemic, in the absence of widespread reliable rapid testing for the diagnosis of COVID-19 infection, include fluid-resistant gown, double gloves, hair cover, and eye protection (goggles or face shield).[59,60] Standard COVID-era respiratory protection includes form-fitting respirators that are able to effectively filter out at least 95% of very

---

Box 4
Ergonomic transabdominal compression

Tips for transabdominal compression
- Focused application in specific beneficial areas
- Reposition patient to improve access
- Keep wrists in neutral position
- Consider forearm use
- Combine with endoscopic techniques

---

small (0.3 micron) particles, called N95 respirators.[60] N95 respirators can be negative pressure, which rely on the user's work of breathing to filter the air, or positive pressure, which supply filtered air to the user with the use of a motorized fan (**Fig. 2**). While respiratory protection is critical to the safety of health care workers, the potential physiologic burden placed on the endoscopy team when using N95 respirators further highlights the need for adequate rest and breaks.

The typical negative pressure N95 respirator is the disposable filtering facepiece respirators (FFPs). An N95 FFP needs to form a tight seal around the user's face, which can be assessed via "fit testing" and uses the wearers' work of breathing to draw air through the masks' nonwoven fibrous filter material to effectively filter out particles. Half-face and full-face elastomeric respirators are alternate negative pressure air-purifying systems that are reusable. These negative pressure respirators may result in an increase in breathing resistance and a reduction in air exchange volume.[61] Continuous, prolonged use of the N95 FFP may result in headaches and reduced tolerance to lighter workloads.[62] When coupled with dehydration, either due to excess perspiration from the burden of PPE or lack of breaks, prolonged use of the N95 may result in headaches, dizziness, and greater distraction from the job. Regular breaks that allow for hydration and fresh air are critical for worker safety and self-care.

Positive pressure respirators, called powered air purifying respirators or "PAPRs", provide an alternative to the N95 FFP. PAPRs generally afford a higher level of respiratory protection than FFP, and the assigned protection factor will depend on if the PAPR is tight or loose fitting, and if it is half or full facepiece, hood or helmet. The loose-fitting PAPR does not require fit testing and is an option for staff who have facial hair or do not pass fit testing with a tight-fitting respirator.[63] As PAPRs provide the user with filtered air using a motorized filter, there is no increased work of breathing with

AIR PURIFYING

TYPES OF RESPIRATORY PROTECTION

Filtering Facepiece Respirators are disposable half facepiece respirators that filter out particles such as dusts, mists, and fumes. They do NOT provide protection against gases and vapors.	**Elastomeric Half Facepiece Respirators** are reusable and have replaceable cartridges or filters. They cover the nose and mouth and provide protection against gases, vapors, or particles when equipped with the appropriate cartridge or filter.	**Elastomeric Full Facepiece Respirators** are reusable and have replaceable canisters, cartridges, or filters. The facepiece covers the face and eyes, which offers eye protection.	**Powered Air-Purifying Respirators (PAPRs)** have a battery-powered blower that pulls air through attached filters, canisters, or cartridges. They provide protection against gases, vapors, or particles, when equipped with the appropriate cartridge, canister, or filter. Loose-fitting PAPRs do not require fit testing and can be used with facial hair.
N95	Elastomer - Half face	Elastomer - Full face	PAPR
NEGATIVE PRESSURE/ Non-powered			POSITIVE PRESSURE

Fig. 2. Types of air purifying respiratory protection, adapted from CDC/NIOSH. The N95 filtering facepiece respirator is a negative pressure respirator. The powered air purifying respirator (PAPR) is a positive pressure respirator. (*From* Centers for Disease Control and Prevention (CDC). Types of Respiratory Protection. Available at: https://www.cdc.gov/coronavirus/2019-ncov/hcp/elastomeric-respirators-strategy/respiratory-protection.html. Accessed December 5, 2020.)

these units. However, the constant noise produced by the PAPR motor can lead to adverse user experiences such as headache, distraction, and difficulty communicating with others.[62]

Many health care workers opt for the N95 FFP over PAPR when considering comfort and ease of communication.[62] The endoscopy team may prefer a PAPR when performing cases on known COVID-positive patients because of the higher assigned protection factor, or when they have experienced adverse effects with prolonged N95 FFP use. Scheduled, frequent rest breaks are essential regardless of the respiratory protection worn.

SUMMARY

Ergonomics affect every aspect of the endoscopy enterprise, from the architectural design of rooms and educational training programs to scheduling and patient handling. Incorporation of ergonomic principles in endoscopy unit design considers patient and staff factors to minimize injury and maximize efficiency. Preprocedure, intraprocedure, and postprocedure areas should aim to deliver patient safety, privacy, and comfort, while also supporting endoscopists and staff with adjustable rooms and effective work flows. During the work day, endoscopists can consider using microbreaks, stretching, and an ergonomic time-out in their practice. As gastroenterology evolves, new technologies may become available to advance endoscopy ergonomics including reevaluation of endoscope instrument design for a diverse population of proceduralists. In the COVID-19 era, it is crucial to preserve ergonomic practices while following new rigorous requirements for PPE. Beyond the endoscopist, a culture of safety during all facets of patient care reduces injury risks and benefits the entire team.

CLINICS CARE POINTS

> - Ergonomics is the science of designing a job to fit the breadth of workers.
>
> - A high prevalence of occupational MSI is well established among endoscopists and gastroenterology nurses and is related to repetitive high force loading in nonneutral postures.
>
> - Team-wide educational initiatives can improve ergonomic awareness.
>
> - Adjustability is key to allow the endoscopy unit staff to maintain neutral body postures and sustain performance during an endoscopy day. Thoughtful design of the endoscopy center's patient care environment that incorporates basic ergonomic principles can optimize efficiency, patient care team satisfaction, and safety.
>
> - Endoscopy staff are advised to pay attention to any symptoms and limit exertion if experiencing pain that may be related to musculoskeletal injury.
>
> - Updated PPE recommendations for performing endoscopy during the COVID pandemic include a fluid resistant gown, double gloves, hair cover, and eye protection (goggles or face shield) in addition to N95 respirators to mitigate airborne spread during endoscopy, which is an aerosol-generating procedure.
>
> - Scheduled, frequent rest breaks are essential.

DISCLOSURE

Dr A.M. Lipowska has nothing to disclose. Dr A.K. Shergill received a research gift from Pentax and is a consultant for Boston Scientific.

REFERENCES

1. Shergill AK, McQuaid KR, Rempel D. Ergonomics and GI endoscopy. Gastrointest Endosc 2009;70(1):145–53.
2. Biomechanics. Musculoskeletal Disorders and the Workplace: Low Back and Upper Extremities. Washington (DC): National Academies Press; 2001.
3. Snedeker JG, Foolen J. Tendon injury and repair - A perspective on the basic mechanisms of tendon disease and future clinical therapy. Acta Biomater 2017; 63:18–36.
4. Yung DE, Banfi T, Ciuti G, et al. Musculoskeletal injuries in gastrointestinal endoscopists: a systematic review. Expert Rev Gastroenterol Hepatol 2017;11(10): 939–47.
5. Morais R, Vilas-Boas F, Pereira P, et al. Prevalence, risk factors and global impact of musculoskeletal injuries among endoscopists: a nationwide European study. Endosc Int Open 2020;8(4):E470–80.
6. Shergill AK, Rempel D, Barr A, et al. Biomechanical risk factors associated with distal upper extremity musculoskeletal disorders in endoscopists performing colonoscopy. Gastrointest Endosc 2021;93(3):704–11.e703.
7. Austin K, Schoenberger H, Sesto M, et al. Musculoskeletal injuries are commonly reported among gastroenterology trainees: results of a national survey. Dig Dis Sci 2019;64(6):1439–47.
8. Zibert K, Singla M, Young PE. Using ergonomics to prevent injuries for the endoscopist. Am J Gastroenterol 2019;114(4):541–3.
9. Siau K, Anderson JT. Ergonomics in endoscopy: Should the endoscopist be considered and trained like an athlete? Endosc Int Open 2019;7(6):E813–5.
10. Khan R, Scaffidi MA, Satchwell J, et al. Impact of a simulation-based ergonomics training curriculum on work-related musculoskeletal injury risk in colonoscopy. Gastrointest Endosc 2020;92(5):1070–80.e1073.
11. Ridtitid W, Cote GA, Leung W, et al. Prevalence and risk factors for musculoskeletal injuries related to endoscopy. Gastrointest Endosc 2015;81(2): 294–302.e294.
12. Piessevaux H. How to predict and achieve success with a very long procedure in an endoscopy unit: Is it time for a break? Endosc Int Open 2019;7(9):E1097–8.
13. Ofori E, Ramai D, John F, et al. Occupation-associated health hazards for the gastroenterologist/endoscopist. Ann Gastroenterol 2018;31(4):448–55.
14. Fahad Ali M, Samarasena J. Implementing ergonomics interventions in the endoscopy suite. Techniques in Gastrointestinal Endoscopy 2019;21(3):159–61.
15. Shergill AK, Harris-Adamson C, Raju GS, et al. Taking Care of You: Ergonomic Essentials for Your Practice (DV074). 2017. Available at:https://learn.asge.org/Public/Catalog/Details.aspx?id=vU4KuIMa78hGWTWg9aRahw%3D%3D&returnurl=%2FUsers%2FUserOnlineCourse.aspx%3FLearningActivityID%3DvU4KuIMa78hGWTWg9aRahw%253d%253d. . Accessed December 5, 2020.
16. Chang MA, Mitchell J, Abbas Fehmi SM. Optimizing ergonomics before endoscopy. VideoGIE 2017;2(7):169.
17. Chang MA, Mitchell J, Abbas Fehmi SM. Optimizing ergonomics during endoscopy. VideoGIE 2017;2(7):170.
18. Chang MA, Mitchell J, Abbas Fehmi SM. Optimizing ergonomics after endoscopy. VideoGIE 2017;2(7):171.
19. Ulrich RS. Effects of interior design on wellness: theory and recent scientific research. J Health Care Inter Des 1991;3:97–109.
20. Jacobs K. Patient Satisfaction by Design. Semin Hear 2016;37(4):316–24.

21. Cappell MS. Injury to endoscopic personnel from tripping over exposed cords, wires, and tubing in the endoscopy suite: a preventable cause of potentially severe workplace injury. Dig Dis Sci 2010;55(4):947–51.
22. Chengular SR, Rodgers SH, Bernard TE. Kodak's Ergonomic Design for People at Work. 2nd ed. Hoboken, NJ: John Wiley & Sons, Inc; 2003.
23. Morl F, Gunther M, Riede JM, et al. Loads distributed in vivo among vertebrae, muscles, spinal ligaments, and intervertebral discs in a passively flexed lumbar spine. Biomech Model Mechanobiol 2020;19(6):2015–47.
24. Padmore CE, Chan AH, Langohr GD, et al. The effect of forearm position on wrist joint biomechanics. J Hand Surg Am 2021;46(5):425.e1–10.
25. Cappell MS. Accidental occupational injuries to endoscopy personnel in a high-volume endoscopy suite during the last decade: mechanisms, workplace hazards, and proposed remediation. Dig Dis Sci 2011;56(2):479–87.
26. Redfern MS, Cham R. The influence of flooring on standing comfort and fatigue. AIHAJ 2000;61(5):700–8.
27. King PM. A comparison of the effects of floor mats and shoe in-soles on standing fatigue. Appl Ergon 2002;33(5):477–84.
28. Kraemer WJ, Volek JS, Bush JA, et al. Influence of compression hosiery on physiological responses to standing fatigue in women. Med Sci Sports Exerc 2000; 32(11):1849–58.
29. Maciel DP, Millen RA, Xavier CA, et al. Musculoskeletal disorder related to the work of doctors who perform medical invasive evaluation. Work 2012;41(Suppl 1):1860–3.
30. Edelman K, Zheng J, Erdmann A, et al. Endoscopy-related musculoskeletal injury in AGA gastroenterologists is common while training in ergonomics is rare. Gastroenterology 2017;152(5):S217.
31. Park AE, Zahiri HR, Hallbeck MS, et al. Intraoperative "Micro Breaks" with targeted stretching enhance surgeon physical function and mental focus: A multi-center cohort study. Ann Surg 2017;265(2):340–6.
32. Shergill AK, Harris-Adamson C. Failure of an engineered system: The gastrointestinal endoscope. Techniques in Gastrointestinal Endoscopy 2019;21(3):116–23.
33. Singla M, Kwok RM, Young PE. Ergonomics of endoscopy. 2017. universe.gi.org/previewpresentation_citation.asp?c514879. Accessed August 8, 2020.
34. Campbell EV 3rd, Muniraj T, Aslanian HR, et al. Musculoskeletal Pain Symptoms and Injuries Among Endoscopists Who Perform ERCP. Dig Dis Sci 2021;66(1): 56–62.
35. Han S, Hammad HT, Wagh MS. High prevalence of musculoskeletal symptoms and injuries in third space endoscopists: an international multicenter survey. Endosc Int Open 2020;8(10):E1481–6.
36. O'Sullivan S, Bridge G, Ponich T. Musculoskeletal injuries among ERCP endoscopists in Canada. Can J Gastroenterol 2002;16(6):369–74.
37. Alexandre D, Prieto M, Beaumont F, et al. Wearing lead aprons in surgical operating rooms: ergonomic injuries evidenced by infrared thermography. J Surg Res 2017;209:227–33.
38. Rothmore P. Lead aprons, radiographers, and discomfort: A pilot study. Journal of Occupational Health and Safety 2002;18(4):357–65.
39. Jowhari F, Hopman WM, Hookey L. A simple ergonomic measure reduces fluoroscopy time during ERCP: A multivariate analysis. Endosc Int Open 2017;5(3): E172–8.
40. Patel N, Darzi A, Teare J. The endoscopy evolution: 'the superscope era'. Frontline Gastroenterol 2015;6(2):101–7.

41. Gonzalez AG, Barrios-Muriel J, Romero-Sanchez F, et al. Ergonomic assessment of a new hand tool design for laparoscopic surgery based on surgeons' muscular activity. Appl Ergon 2020;88:103161.

42. Tung KD, Shorti RM, Downey EC, et al. The effect of ergonomic laparoscopic tool handle design on performance and efficiency. Surg Endosc 2015;29(9):2500–5.

43. Drysdale SA. The incidence of upper extremity injuries in endoscopy nurses. Gastroenterol Nurs 2007;30(3):187–92.

44. Drysdale S. The incidence of upper extremity injuries in Canadian endoscopy nurses. Gastroenterol Nurs 2011;34(1):26–33.

45. Drysdale SA. The incidence of upper extremity injuries in endoscopy nurses working in the United States. Gastroenterol Nurs 2013;36(5):329–38.

46. Murty M. Musculoskeletal disorders in endoscopy nursing. Gastroenterol Nurs 2010;33(5):354–61.

47. Drysdale SA. The incidence of neck and back injuries in endoscopy nurses working in the United States of America. Gastroenterol Nurs 2014;37(2):187–8.

48. Occupational Safety and Health Administration. Safe Patient Handling [Website]. 2020. Available at: https://www.osha.gov/dsg/hospitals/patient_handling.html. Accessed November 14, 2020.

49. The National Institute for Occupational Safety and Health (NIOSH). Safe Patient Handling and Mobility (SPHM) 2020. Available at: https://www.cdc.gov/niosh/topics/safepatient/default.html. Accessed November 14, 2020.

50. Committee AT, Walsh CM, Umar SB, et al. Colonoscopy core curriculum. Gastrointest Endosc 2021;93(2):297–304.

51. Prechel JA, Sedlack RE, Harreld FA, et al. Looping and abdominal pressure: A visual guide to a successful colonoscopy. Gastroenterol Nurs 2015;38(4):289–94, quiz 295-286.

52. Yu GQ, Huang XM, Li HY, et al. Use of an abdominal obstetric binder in colonoscopy: A randomized, prospective trial. J Gastroenterol Hepatol 2018;33(7):1365–9.

53. Nishizawa T, Suzuki H, Higuchi H, et al. Effects of Encircled Abdominal Compression Device in Colonoscopy: A Meta-Analysis. J Clin Med 2019;9(1).

54. Crockett SD, Cirri HO, Kelapure R, et al. Use of an Abdominal Compression Device in Colonoscopy: A Randomized, Sham-Controlled Trial. Clin Gastroenterol Hepatol 2016;14(6):850–7.e853.

55. SGNA. Position Statement: Ergonomics in the Gastroenterology Setting. 2014. Available at: https://www.sgna.org/Portals/0/Education/PDF/Position-Statements/SGNA_PositionStatement_Ergonomics_2014.pdf.

56. Centers for Disease Control and Prevention. 2020. Available at:https://www.cdc.gov/coronavirus/2019-ncov/prevent-getting-sick/how-covid-spreads.html. . Accessed December 30, 2020.

57. Soetikno R, Teoh AYB, Kaltenbach T, et al. Considerations in performing endoscopy during the COVID-19 pandemic. Gastrointest Endosc 2020;92(1):176–83.

58. Cheung KS, Hung IFN, Chan PPY, et al. Gastrointestinal Manifestations of SARS-CoV-2 Infection and Virus Load in Fecal Samples From a Hong Kong Cohort: Systematic Review and Meta-analysis. Gastroenterology 2020;159(1):81–95.

59. American Society for Gastrointestinal Endoscopy. Available at:https://www.asge.org/home/resources/key-resources/covid-19-asge-updates-for-members/joint-gastroenterology-society-message-covid-19-use-of-personal-protective-equipment-in-gi-endoscopy. Accessed December 30, 2020.

60. Sultan S, Lim JK, Altayar O, et al. AGA rapid recommendations for gastrointestinal procedures during the COVID-19 pandemic. Gastroenterology 2020; 159(2):739–58.e734.
61. Lee HP, Wang de Y. Objective assessment of increase in breathing resistance of N95 respirators on human subjects. Ann Occup Hyg 2011;55(8):917–21.
62. Centers for Disease Control and Prevention. The Physiological Burden of Prolonged PPE Use on Healthcare Workers during Long Shifts. 2020. Available at:https://blogs.cdc.gov/niosh-science-blog/2020/06/10/ppe-burden/. . Accessed December 30, 2020.
63. The National Institute for Occupational Safety and Health (NIOSH). A Guide to Air-Purifying Respirators. 2018. Available at: https://www.cdc.gov/niosh/docs/2018-176/default.html. Accessed December 30, 2020.

Endoscopic Supply Chain Management and Optimization

Ji Seok Park, MD, Sunguk N. Jang, MD*

KEYWORDS

- Supply chain management • Endoscopic practice • Endoscopy
- Multidisciplinary endoscopic device committee • Group purchasing organization

KEY POINTS

- To improve the value-based care in endoscopic procedures, supply chain management, and optimization is of paramount importance.
- Creating a multidisciplinary supply chain management team, such as multidisciplinary endoscopic device committee (MEDC), in conjunction with participating in group purchasing organization can optimize the supply chain management.
- The three essential components of MEDC are physicians, clinical administration, and institutional supply chain.
- The three important tasks of MEDC are clinical care–aligned product acquisition, review of meaningful use of products, and utilization of guidelines creation.

INTRODUCTION

The United States spends more on health care than any other country, with cost approaching 18% of the national gross domestic product and $3.6 trillion in 2018.[1,2] Up to 25% of health care spending is attributed to waste, and continuous efforts have been made to make the health care system more efficient.[3] In 2010, the Institute of Medicine identified six categories of potential source of waste in the US health care spending, including pricing failure from variability and inflation in pricing of devices and procedures.[4] A portion of high health care spending and health care waste comes from the multibillion dollar gastrointestinal endoscopic device market as endoscopy is a procedural specialty that incurs significant cost through its high usage of disposable accessories.[5] Thus, supply chain management in endoscopy is of paramount importance in improving the value-based care because it can identify areas of cost savings in device procurement.[6] In addition, as new technology refines

Department of Gastroenterology, Hepatology and Nutrition, Cleveland Clinic, 9500 Euclid Avenue, Cleveland, OH 44195, USA
* Corresponding author.
E-mail address: jangs@ccf.org

Gastrointest Endoscopy Clin N Am 31 (2021) 671–679
https://doi.org/10.1016/j.giec.2021.05.004
1052-5157/21/© 2021 Elsevier Inc. All rights reserved.

giendo.theclinics.com

previous endoscopic procedures and creates new ones, optimizing the value assessment through a well-established supply chain system can be deemed more significant.[7] With this, we have created a MEDC for our large and dynamic academic health system to optimize supply chain.

NATURE OF THE PROBLEM

Traditionally, endoscopic device procurement is centered around the personal relationship between a device sales representative and physicians. After physicians assess the product through trials and the product is deemed competitive by the user, the endoscopy center manager makes an acquisition request. While this model has been in place for some time, this model of purchasing has several limitations as there is an absence of centralized regulation or guidelines. First of all, there is a lack of uniformed product performance assessment when the purchase is made. Second, there is a risk of purchasing an inappropriate amount of product or having multiple items with similar functionality. Finally, it is difficult to monitor its utilization and maintain an appropriate supply par level in inventory. To resolve these limitations, a centralized and integrative MEDC can play an important role. Furthermore, this committee can prevent any personal relationships from overriding an objective and transparent endoscopic device procurement process.

The inclusion and empowerment of physicians in an endoscopic supply chain committee is vital to its optimal performance. Creating a centralized "wholesale" purchasing system without physicians who understand the procedures and pertinent equipment utilization can lead to undesirable outcomes in multiple facets. In Canadian health care system for instance, the involvement of physicians in the purchasing process has been limited in their endoscopy units. This is primarily because purchasing and organizing the budget is performed through the hospital's executive management and a regional administrative service.[8] In British Columbia, there is a centralized purchasing agency known as Health Shared Services British Columbia (HSSBC), which acts on behalf of all British Columbia health networks to negotiate with individual vendors to achieve a consistent, discounted pricing as well as a reliable supply chain. In this setting, a group of researchers conducted a study to investigate the operating performance of a large GI clinic. The aim of the study was to examine the caseload breakdown, gain a better understanding of the characteristics that impacted the budgetary performance of the GI clinic, and formulate recommendations to encourage better utilization of available resources. The findings showed that approximately half of all expenditure at this clinic was cost-associated with supplies and consumables. Initially, the statement of operations appeared to have appropriately recorded expenditures by using different equipment categories, which directly mirrored the HSSBC catalog of products. However, upon closer scrutiny, multiple critical miscategorizations were discovered. For example, endoscopic ultrasound fine-needle aspiration needles, metal esophageal stents, and endoscopic retrograde cholangiopancreatography (ERCP) guidewires were placed under the category "Enteral feedings". The authors pointed out that this miscategorization makes it impossible to obtain an accurate accounting of supplies and consumables spending, preventing precise assessment of utilization. This miscategorization was deemed preventable if physicians, who understand the endoscopic procedures, were involved in the centralized supply chain system.

A successful example of health care value improvement through clinical community and supply chain collaboration was also reported from a large academic healthy system in the United States.[9] Johns Hopkins Medicine launched a system-wide supply chain initiative to manage financial challenges and to decrease waste in 2016. The supply chain management team renegotiated contracts with vendors, optimized the procurement process, and partnered with clinical communities involving physicians who provided valuable input on the quality of different products under consideration. The management team's focused efforts to reduce supply costs included spine surgery, joint replacement, and blood transfusion management. Upon assessment, the team noticed that their health system, comprised of different hospitals, was failing to work in a coordinated manner to take advantage of their "health system" unity when negotiating with vendors. The clinical communities and supply chain management team decided to form a GPO to leverage cost saving during renegotiation, along with using a vendor price-capping model. As a result, the health system saved multi-million dollars in device procurement while maintaining quality as a priority.

Components and Responsibilities of the Multidisciplinary Endoscopic Device Committee

One of the core components of MEDC is physician integration. This helps to develop strategy and define the value of the product in executing value-based purchase decisions. In health care, value is defined as the patient's health outcomes over cost, and the two critical components of an outcome are efficacy and safety.[10] Also, MEDC begins with identifying and recruiting two other core components: clinical administration and institutional supply chain (**Fig. 1**). The core objectives of the MEDC are (i) product purchase in alignment with the portfolio of clinical services provided; (ii) reduction in cost variation and wasteful spending across the organization; (iii) formulating evidence-based outcome to improve the quality of practice; and (iv) encouraging problem solution with team-based approach (**Fig. 2**).

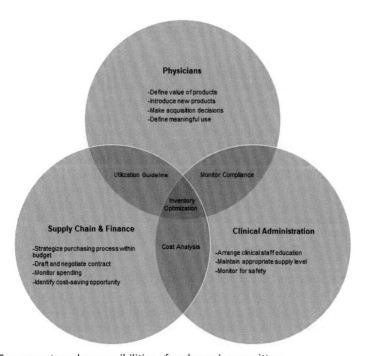

Fig. 1. Components and responsibilities of endoscopic committees.

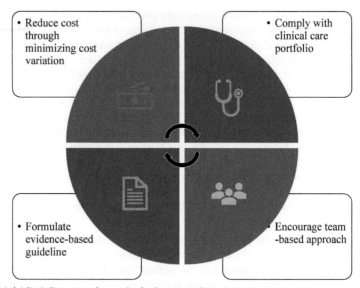

Fig. 2. Multidisciplinary endoscopic device committee core concept.

The physicians in the committee serve as team leaders with the four responsibilities. First, to define the value of the product, they are expected to provide clinical opinions and review efficacy and safety data during the product trial. Second, when new technology or product has the possibility of improving patient outcomes, these physicians identify and introduce new products. Third, they participate in and lead the product-acquisition decision-making process. Finally, they generate a practice guideline to define meaningful use of the product and aid clinical administration in monitoring systemic compliance.

Working closely with a finance administrator, the supply chain representatives are responsible for facilitating and prioritizing the purchasing process within the limits of the budget; negotiating with device vendors regarding the details of purchases; drafting contracts for physician leadership to review; calculating financial impact before the purchase and keep track of actual spending attributed to specific products; and identifying any cost-saving opportunities by analyzing product utilization. They are also tasked to provide regularly scheduled updates in the outcomes of the committee's endeavor to maintain financial transparency and sustain motivation.

The clinical administrators, working with nurse managers and inventory managers, arrange education for nurses and endoscopy technicians on proper utilization of endoscopic devices, maintain the desired par level, and generate reports for the committee on product usage and safety/adverse events related to the product. They should also serve as a conduit of communication between vendor, physicians, and nursing staff if concern for improper utilization arises.

TASKS OF THE MULTIDISCIPLINARY ENDOSCOPIC DEVICE COMMITTEE
Clinical Care–Aligned Product Acquisition

An open-access product-evaluation platform called MedApproved is used at our institution. Using this platform, a physician can submit a new endoscopic device/technology for peer-based trial and evaluation (**Fig. 3**). When a request is submitted, MEDC members are briefed on its utility and potential benefit by a "physician champion."

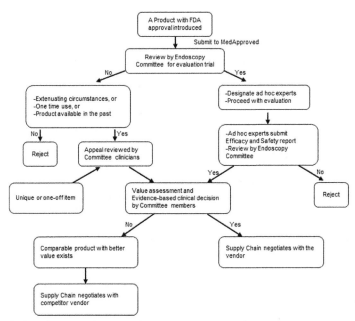

Fig. 3. Multidisciplinary endoscopic device committee product process acquisition.

Then, the clinicians on the committee review the product and decide on whether to proceed with an evaluation trial. MEDC also identifies *ad hoc* experts to participate in the trial because this is helpful for the product vendors to agree on providing the product at "no-cost" basis during the evaluation period. When the product is deemed not appropriate for an evaluation trial, it is rejected by the committee unless it has extenuating circumstances (ie, the previous version of the device is well-known to the committee, and the new version has only a few additional features, or the device has an available credible report on efficacy and safety and has proven to be more effective than current devices, or rarely, when there are no other options because of changes in the supply chain), it is only for one-time use, or the product was presented to the committee in the past. The product without an evaluation trial is reviewed by the committee clinicians who assess its value and make an evidence-based clinical decision with other committee members.

For the product that undergoes an evaluation trial and whose efficacy and safety are deemed acceptable by the reviewers, the committee proceeds to assess the product's value, where the cost of the product is compared with similar items that may already be in the inventory. When the product is deemed a better choice, and there are no potential conflicts with an existing contract, the decision is made to purchase the item. Afterward, the supply chain representatives draft a contract and negotiate with device vendors based on a projected market share and duration. When there are potential conflicts with an existing contract or when there is a possibility of reducing cost of existing product, supply chain representatives can renegotiate with a competitor vendor. Importantly, a significant cost saving during negotiation can occur at a health care institution that belongs to a large GPO.

When an item is considered unique ("carved-out"), clinicians assess its value based on whether the product aligns with the spectrum of clinical services that the organization provides and make a decision consulting with other committee members.

Review of Meaningful Use

There are two important functions of the product utilization report provided by the supply chain during regularly occurring meetings. It is essential to "declutter" the inventory by removing unused or rarely used items when new products are added to the system. The initial draft is formulated based on inventory utilization logs generated by inventory managers. Then, this is passed on to supply chain representatives. Working closely with endoscopic operation of the organization, the MEDC will decide whether to retain or remove products. It is recommended that the committee will identify the experts who frequently perform the procedures and ascertain their opinion before the final decision.

Second, analytics on cost per case will monitor for any concerning trend regarding a particular device usage within the organization. Before embarking on the project, it is critical to inform the intent and process to the stakeholders (including physicians). For optimal impact, it is recommended to start the review with a high-volume therapeutic procedure (eg, colonoscopy with polypectomy) and the costliest procedure (eg, ERCP with metal stent placement). In addition, analytics can identify any physician whose product utilization is not aligned with that of others in the organization. If the physician's product utilization varies from other users, the committee can remind and re-educate the physician on proper use of the product. In our experience, the need for corrective action can often be avoided when a physician of concern is addressed with transparent and standardized metrics.

Utilization of Guidelines Creation

MEDC can also contribute to the quality-of-care assessment and improvement. It is easier to assess procedural performance when product utilization within an institution is unified. The institution's outcomes data and analysis can be helpful in creating an evidence-based product utilization guideline. It is beneficial to choose an impactful endoscopic procedure, such as endoscopic hemostasis, that lacks an institutional guideline and displays significant heterogeneity in product utilization (eg, the use of hemostatic powder during endoscopic hemostasis). Then, the aggregation of data for the product utilization and procedural outcomes is important. Reviewing existing, pertinent literature on the subject matter is a requisite in minimizing potential institutional bias. The final device utilization guideline should contain clear numeric data-based recommendations so that users can follow it easily and the compliance can be objectively assessed.

A good example of guideline utilization by multidisciplinary supply chain committee can be seen in Johns Hopkins Medicine's effort to reduce supply cost in blood management.[9] Blood transfusion is the most commonly used procedure in US hospitals[11] and has shown a wide variation of its use in practice.[12] Based on the blood utilization cost data, the supply chain committee involving physicians noticed the variation in practice among hospitals and providers in the absence of outcome variability.[9] Thus, the evidence-based health system–wide transfusion guidelines were made and distributed to hospitals along with multiple education events across the health system.[9] The events emphasized the variation in transfusion practice according to hemoglobin trigger thresholds, and the known risks and adverse events of transfusion, along with the opportunity to reduce these risks as well as costs. This effort not only reduced the annual transfusion cost by 1.2 million dollars[9] but also contributed to quality-of-care assessment and improvement by creating and reinforcing appropriate guidelines.

Challenges and Problem Solutions with Team-Based Approach

In our organization, a product quality issue arose during a conversion process. To troubleshoot, a physician champion met with the vendor along with the supply chain team to review the quality issue. The vendor proposed a detailed corrective action plan, which eventually included a completely new production facility and re-evaluation. Once changes were applied and issues corrected, MEDC carefully restarted the conversion process while closely monitoring performance.

Group Purchasing Organization

The benefit of the multidisciplinary supply chain committee can be maximized in conjunction with GPO. A GPO is an entity which aggregates purchasing volume of health care providers to save costs by getting quantity discounts from manufacturers and distributors.[13] By participating in a GPO, an organization can save significant amount of supply cost. In addition, GPO often provides product utilization guidelines that are physician-driven and evidence-based. The guidelines not only reduce supply variation but also delivers clinical care alignment. For example, a surgical mesh guideline for ventral hernia repair was made and distributed to health care providers from a GPO that our organization participates in. The guideline included mesh selection algorithm according to hernia's degree of contamination (ie, clean, clean/contaminated, contaminated, and dirty) to standardize the selection process. By using the same type of mesh in identical clinical situations, the guideline implementation enabled quality measures in performance of every physician who participated in GPO. The medical advisory board is responsible for the creation and distribution of guidelines, which is a council comprised of physicians that oversee and monitor GPO from the perspective of member input and clinical outcome. The council meet twice per year to review meaningful use of each product, feedback from members, and any relevant health care events.

Future Endoscopic Supply Chains

As these recommendations are established in a large academic institution, it may have to be applied differently in ambulatory surgical centers (ASCs). In small endoscopic centers where there is a scarcity of infrastructure in finance administrator and supply chain management, physicians can play more important roles in the supply chain management.

Furthermore, small endoscopic centers will benefit from moving from the traditional "batch production model" to a new "continuous flow model," which is already being implemented in other industries.[14] This continuous processing model has substantial opportunities in inventory reduction compared with a large batch model as the new model is a more demand-responsive end-to-end supply chain. With the continuous processing supply chain, the volume options for "minimum order quantities," which has been a key criterion in traditional supply chain design, become potentially unconstrained. In addition, continuous processing can more easily improve quality of endoscopic device, through continuous process control and enforcing process conditions at a microlevel, which has a fundamental impact on development process on quality and on supply.

Another future supply chain implementation path is the use of 3D printing systems.[14] Three-dimensional printing is a process where objects can be fabricated layer by layer, or part by part, allowing computer design and easy customization of products. The ultimate outcome would be the development of software-only manufacturing workflows whereby the physical system could be configured electronically. Endoscopic centers will be able to "print" a new endoscopic device with appropriate amount for its usage.

SUMMARY

With the goal of providing cost-effective endoscopic services across the organization, MEDC is a new concept of acquiring, monitoring, and leveraging endoscopic product purchase and utilization. In our organization, MEDC achieved annual savings of approximately $0.6 million (9%) from endoscopic device budget. The limitation of our recommendations is that these were established and implemented in a large academic institution, thus they may have to be applied differently in ASCs. To summarize, in conjunction with GPO, MEDC suggests a model to optimize the endoscopy supply chain management by meeting the demands of quality health care at an affordable price.

CLINICS CARE POINTS

- The cost of endoscopic disposable devices remains a significant financial burden to any health care facility.
- The optimal approach to cost saving for endoscopic disposable devices is achieved by a multidisciplinary team comprising clinicians, administrative staffs, and supply chain representatives.
- Value-based approach, where value is defined as outcome over cost, allows clinicians to be the key decision-maker in the purchasing process of endoscopic devices.
- The clinicians involved in health care product acquisition process should be well versed in pricing and negotiation process.

DISCLOSURE

The authors have nothing to disclose.

REFERENCES

1. Papanicolas I, Woskie LR, Jha AK. Health care spending in the United States and other high-income countries. JAMA 2018;319(10):1024–39.
2. Hartman M, Martin AB, Benson J, et al. National Health Care Spending In 2018: Growth Driven By Accelerations In Medicare And Private Insurance Spending: US health care spending increased 4.6 percent to reach $3.6 trillion in 2018, a faster growth rate than that of 4.2 percent in 2017 but the same rate as in 2016. Health Aff 2020;39(1):8–17.
3. Shrank WH, Rogstad TL, Parekh N. Waste in the US health care system: estimated costs and potential for savings. JAMA 2019;322(15):1501–9.
4. Institute of Medicine Roundtable on Evidence-Based M. The National Academies Collection: Reports funded by National Institutes of Health. In: Yong PL, Saunders RS, Olsen L, editors. The healthcare imperative: lowering costs and improving outcomes: workshop series Summary. Washington (DC): National Academies Press (US) Copyright © 2010, National Academy of Sciences.; 2010.
5. Petersen BT. Advantages of disposable endoscopic accessories. Gastrointest Endosc Clin N Am 2000;10(2):341–8.
6. Jang S, Jones B, Vargo J. Supply chain management for endoscopic practice. Am J Gastroenterol 2019;114(9):1403–6.
7. Croffie J, Carpenter S, Chuttani R, et al. ASGE technology status evaluation report: disposable endoscopic accessories. Gastrointest Endosc 2005;62(4):477–9.
8. Lee SS, Enns R. The hidden realities of endocopy unit budgeting. Can J Gastroenterol Hepatol 2014;28(11):619–20.

9. Ishii L, Demski R, Lee KK, et al. Improving healthcare value through clinical community and supply chain collaboration. Paper presented at: Healthcare 2017.
10. Porter ME. What is value in health care. N Engl J Med 2010;363(26):2477–81.
11. Pfuntner A, Wier L, Stocks C. Most frequent procedures performed in US hospitals, 2010: Statistical Brief# 149 2006: Healthcare Cost and Utilization Project (HCUP) Statistical Briefs [Internet].
12. Frank SM, Savage WJ, Rothschild JA, et al. Variability in blood and blood component utilization as assessed by an anesthesia information management system. Anesthesiology 2012;117(1):99–106.
13. Ahmadi A, Pishvaee MS, Heydari M. How group purchasing organisations influence healthcare-product supply chains? An analytical approach. J Oper Res Soc 2019;70(2):280–93.
14. Srai JS, Badman C, Krumme M, et al. Future supply chains enabled by continuous processing—Opportunities and challenges. May 20–21, 2014 Continuous Manufacturing Symposium. J Pharm Sci 2015;104(3):840–9.

The Role of the Gastrointestinal Hospitalist in Optimizing Endoscopic Operations

Edward Sun, MD, MBA[a],*, Michelle L. Hughes, MD[b],
Sarah Enslin, PA-C[c], Kathy Bull-Henry, MD[d], Vivek Kaul, MD[c],
Glenn D. Littenberg, MD, MACP[e,1]

KEYWORDS

- Hospitalist • GI hospitalist • Endoscopic operations • Optimizing endoscopy
- Inpatient endoscopy • Outpatient endoscopy • Hospital outpatient department
- Endoscopy efficiency

KEY POINTS

- Through improved interdisciplinary care coordination, gastroenterology (GI) hospitalists can provide more efficient inpatient care, reducing delays and barriers to endoscopy.
- GI hospitalist models are increasingly incorporating advanced practice providers to further enhance inpatient clinical care.
- In light of increasing demand for procedures, decreasing office reimbursements, and high fixed costs of endoscopy, the GI hospitalist model improves outpatient endoscopy efficiency.
- There is a growing opportunity for interventional endoscopy–trained fellows to explore careers as GI hospitalists.

 Video content accompanies this article at http://www.giendo.theclinics.com.

Dr V. Kaul and Dr G.D. Littenberg contributed equally to this article and should both be acknowledged as senior authors.

[a] Division of Gastroenterology & Hepatology, Department of Medicine, Stony Brook University Hospital, 101 Nicolls Road, HSC T17-060, Stony Brook, NY 11794-8173, USA; [b] Department of Medicine, Section of Digestive Diseases, Yale School of Medicine, PO Box 208019, New Haven, CT 06520, USA; [c] Division of Gastroenterology and Hepatology, University of Rochester Medical Center, 601 Elmwood Avenue, Box 646, Rochester, NY 14642, USA; [d] Endoscopy Unit, Johns Hopkins Bayview Hospital, Johns Hopkins Medicine, 4940 Eastern Avenue, Building A, 5th Floor, Baltimore, MD 21224, USA; [e] inSite Digestive Healthcare, Pasadena, CA, USA
[1] Present address: 630 South Raymond Avenue, Pasadena, CA 91105.
* Corresponding author.
E-mail address: edward.sun@stonybrookmedicine.edu

THE ROLE OF THE GASTROINTESTINAL HOSPITALIST

Dr Edward Sun outlines the areas discussed in this article regarding the role of the gastrointestinal/gastroenterology (GI) hospitalist in optimizing endoscopic operations in Video 1.

Over the last few decades, the practice of GI has evolved rapidly on many fronts. In particular, endoscopic operations have seen dramatic improvements and refinement in increasing patient access, quality of care, and efficiency. These trends are in no small part caused by advancements in technology, a better understanding of operational efficiencies, and the pressures of decreasing reimbursement and increasing costs.

More recently, the role of the GI hospitalist has made a significant impact on endoscopic practice. This article describes the GI hospitalist model and its role in improving patient satisfaction, enhancing quality of care, and introducing efficiencies in endoscopic operations. Specific attributes of the GI hospitalist model also discussed include improved communication and interdisciplinary coordination, timely access to care, and better transitions for posthospital outpatient follow-up care of the patient.

The impact of the GI hospitalist model on endoscopic operations is examined in 3 areas: inpatient endoscopy, outpatient endoscopy, and the hospital outpatient department (HOPD). The challenges and opportunities associated with a GI hospitalist model and supporting a GI hospitalist team are reviewed. Special consideration is given to the role of the GI hospitalist in relation to advanced endoscopy. In addition, the role of the GI hospitalist in endoscopy quality measurement and the financial implications for the GI practice overall given the current movement toward value-based care are also explored.

This article highlights the multiple ways a GI hospitalist model can contribute to progress in the practice of endoscopy. As GI practices and endoscopic operations continue to evolve, the GI hospitalist paradigm represents a transformational opportunity for improving endoscopic quality and efficiency, and, ultimately, the patient experience. Greater awareness of this model and tailoring it to fit the needs of the individual GI practice or endoscopy unit will be key to practice sustainability and growth.

THE GASTROENTEROLOGY HOSPITALIST AND INPATIENT ENDOSCOPY

Dr Michelle Hughes defines the GI hospitalist model and its impact on inpatient endoscopy in Video 2.

Over the past 2 decades, the hospitalist model grew in prevalence as practitioners increasingly moved away from providing concurrent inpatient and outpatient care.[1] Following the success of the hospitalist model in the practice of internal medicine,[2] various other specialties have established dedicated inpatient-care practices: neurology,[3,4] obstetrics and gynecology,[5] and more recently GI.[6] At its core, the GI hospitalist model is structured around a gastroenterologist who provides on-site care to hospital-based patients. For the duration that GI hospitalists are assigned inpatient service, they do not have outpatient office hours or outpatient procedures. As such, their time and attention can be devoted exclusively to providing timely, high-quality consultative services to hospitalized patients.

From discussions with GI hospitalists across the United States, many variations on the GI hospitalist model exist. The role of the GI hospitalist remains in an early stage of evolution and the lack of a well-defined model reflects the marked variation in not only specific GI practice structure and needs but also in health system demands, financial constraints, and provider preferences. Although most GI hospitalist models consist of 1 or 2 inpatient gastroenterologists blocked for alternating inpatient tours of 1 or

2 weeks, some GI practices employ 2 or more GI hospitalists working in parallel or in collaboration, either in rotating roles or covering different sites. Depending on the needs of the hospital or health system, 1 GI hospitalist may staff consults and the other remains dedicated to performing inpatient procedures generated from those consults. Additional GI hospitalists may be employed to staff a primary GI inpatient service caring for patients with common conditions such as gastrointestinal bleeding, inflammatory bowel disease, and decompensated cirrhosis. Other systems may use a full-time GI hospitalist to provide consult and procedure services during the day but still rely on voluntary or on-call staff at night. This strategy preserves continuity for the inpatient service, reduces disruption to outpatient provider schedules, and mitigates risk of burnout for both the GI hospitalists and their outpatient colleagues.

The week-to-week schedule of a GI hospitalist varies as well. Some GI hospitalist models are structured around a Monday through Friday schedule with alternating off weeks, whereas others rely on a full 7-day coverage system. Most GI hospitalists have nonworking or noninpatient weeks woven into their schedules with specific amounts of time and out-of-hospital responsibilities varying significantly between systems. Coverage of after-hours or on-call responsibilities is also highly variable from practice to practice, with some GI hospitalists enjoying a reduced frequency of on-call coverage compared with other members of their practice. These details often depend on balancing the needs of the GI practice with those of the hospital and the practice, accounting for the size and acuity level of the care center and the volume of inpatient versus outpatient patients.

THE GASTROENTEROLOGY HOSPITALIST TEAM

Sarah Enslin describes the role of the advanced practice provider on the GI hospitalist team in Video 3.

GI hospitalist models are increasingly incorporating advanced practice providers (APPs: physician assistants or nurse practitioners) to further enhance inpatient clinical care. The role of the APP may vary, with some models using APPs solely in the hospital and others delegating both inpatient and outpatient responsibilities to their APPs. As part of the inpatient team, APPs help the gastroenterologist maximize endoscopy time by performing initial consultations and follow-up care, ordering and interpreting diagnostic studies, and providing follow-up recommendations and communication with primary teams. The APP's responsibilities may include helping primary teams optimize patients before endoscopic procedures with great attention and sensitivity to issues that may delay endoscopy.[7] These duties may involve patient education, pharmacologic management (eg, antithrombotic agents, diabetic medications), discussion with other specialists (eg, obtaining cardiac clearance), obtaining consent from the patient or their health care proxy, and verifying that preprocedure transfusions have been completed. In addition, APPs can provide enhanced oversight to primary teams when bowel preps are found to be suboptimal, thus salvaging inpatient colonoscopies that would have otherwise been canceled. APPs can directly improve endoscopy unit workflow by performing follow-up on patients postprocedure while the gastroenterologist is starting the next procedure, including postprocedure charting, order entry, communication with patients and family members, and updating other specialists or primary teams regarding procedure results and recommendations. They may also provide specialized education to patients before and even after discharge. Some APPs may perform in a hybrid role, with 1 or more outpatient clinics. Seeing patients quickly postdischarge can reduce length of stay and improve patient outcomes and patient satisfaction.[8]

Additional team members can also contribute to the successful inpatient GI service by addressing specific barriers to care. A nurse navigator can help coordinate procedures, liaise with medical teams, identify and correct preprocedural issues involving medical optimization or poor preps, or coordinate care in the case of conflicting or overlapping tests or procedures such as hemodialysis or imaging studies that could lead to delays in endoscopy. They can also provide essential services once procedures or consults are completed by focusing on patient education and transitions to outpatient care facilitating follow-up procedures and clinic appointments. Whether on a busy consult service where additional support is required or in a smaller practice where demand may not be great enough to support funding of an APP, a nurse navigator can help reduce burden on GI hospitalists without adding substantial costs of hiring a licensed independent practitioner. Another team member that can help optimize the workflow of a GI hospitalist team is a dedicated patient transporter. In many systems, delays in transport lead to significant strain on endoscopy unit efficiency and can lead to procedure cancelations. Tasking an endoscopy tech or nurse on a just-in-time basis for transport duties can significantly improve endoscopy unit throughput, thereby allowing more procedures to be completed each day.

INPATIENT ENDOSCOPY

Perhaps the most immediate effect the GI hospitalist model has on endoscopic operations is with inpatient endoscopy. The demand for gastrointestinal specialty consultation[9] and endoscopic services for hospitalized patients has been increasing.[10] Furthermore, with greater outpatient management of chronic illnesses, the average severity of illness, risk of mortality, and case mix index for patients admitted to the hospital have escalated impressively.[11] Patients presenting to the emergency room increasingly are older,[12] sicker, and more complex.[13] The number of patients admitted for gastrointestinal bleeding, for example, has increased with the increase in use of anticoagulation and antiplatelet therapy for cardiac disease.[14,15] In addition, time-pressured medical decisions often need to be made despite incomplete information (with inadequate histories and a lack of complete records). These characteristics inherent to the inpatient GI consult service make it particularly challenging for gastroenterologists who are concurrently managing busy outpatient practices. The traditional model therefore has the potential to delay access to care for inpatients as well as contributing to physician burnout.

The hospitalist role is particularly suited for those physicians who have a personality and temperament that thrives in high-intensity situations managing high-acuity patients. It spurs GI hospitalists to gain aptitude and expertise in managing critically ill patients on a regular basis. The paucity of data surrounding the impact of GI hospitalists on quality of care likely reflects a field still in development rather than a lack of true benefit. In the few publications to date, GI hospitalists have been shown to have some ability to decrease time to upper endoscopy for urgent indications as well as shorten length of stay and cost of admission for upper gastrointestinal bleeding. A retrospective cohort study conducted at Columbia University Medical Center in New York found that a GI hospitalist system was associated with a statistically significant decreased time from GI consultation to upper endoscopy in patients evaluated urgently, after adjusting for sedation, weekend consultation, and weekly procedure volume (14.0 vs 23.8 hours; ratio = 0.55; 95% confidence interval, 0.33–0.91; $P = .02$).[16] Expanding on experience from other procedural specialties where inpatients pose a significant challenge in acuity and complexity, hospitalist models have been shown to decrease time to consultation and to procedure, shorten length of stay, improve trainee supervision, decrease procedural complications, and improve outcomes.[17–19]

GI hospitalists must be proficient in performing complex endoscopic procedures and managing GI emergencies such as bleeding, foreign body impactions, and sigmoid volvulus.[20] Familiarity with clinical care algorithms and the tools to treat such conditions can improve efficiency in endoscopy with more streamlined approaches and result in more timely care to patients with improved outcomes and patient satisfaction.

It is commonly accepted that inpatient endoscopy, in general, is less efficient than outpatient endoscopy. Hospitalized patients are typically sicker, more complex, and demand greater consideration and time with all aspects of endoscopy from anesthesia assessment to the procedure and immediate postprocedure care. Moreover, room turnover time, and the time interval between successive inpatient procedures, can be affected by many factors, including those unrelated to the endoscopy unit.[21] Arrival to endoscopy may be delayed depending on the floor nurse's responsibilities and availability of patient transport. Procedures may be canceled for any number of reasons, including patient clinical instability, improperly timed laboratory tests, failure to remain nil by mouth, or neglect to hold anticoagulation. GI hospitalists must become adept at navigating their complex hospital systems and learn to preempt the many pitfalls that threaten to delay inpatient procedures. From managing poor bowel preps to electrolyte repletion, from under-resuscitation to obtaining appropriate informed consent in cases involving a patient without capacity, experienced GI hospitalists can introduce great efficiency in inpatient endoscopy practice. GI hospitalists are also more likely to have developed close professional relationships with general medicine and surgical hospitalists and their APPs. These close working relationships can result in patients getting more efficient care with fewer delays and unnecessary tests by increasing communication and establishing familiarity of team expectations and procedural needs. This positive impact on interdisciplinary care and coordination cannot be overemphasized.

GI hospitalists can also bring efficiency to the endoscopy schedule by gaining familiarity and developing close working relationships with members of their own units. This includes the anesthesiologists that rotate through the inpatient endoscopy unit, nursing staff, unit managers, and supply personnel. With regard to anesthesia, frequent collaboration with anesthesia staff on high-risk, high-acuity cases results in greater trust as well as mutual understanding of each other's clinical needs and abilities. This approach can result in fewer cancelations and improved risk stratification and case selection for inpatient procedures and the site of performance (operating room vs endoscopy suite). Working closely with endoscopy unit staff on complex cases also lends itself to improved efficiency. GI hospitalists who build relationships with unit staff can better identify areas for improvement, whether related to staff training, supply issues, or room turnover, thereby further improving care and reducing barriers to endoscopy.

OUTPATIENT ENDOSCOPY

Dr Vivek Kaul describes the positive impact of the GI hospitalist model on outpatient endoscopic operations in Video 4.

Outpatient endoscopy is typically performed at an ambulatory endoscopy center (AEC; office endoscopy) or ambulatory surgery center (ASC). The increasing demand for endoscopic procedures and increasing cost of equipment, with only incremental increases in endoscopy reimbursement rates, make maximizing endoscopic efficiency vital to sustaining the financial success of the outpatient GI practice.

Various trends are likely to increase the demand for endoscopic services. These trends include lowering the colorectal cancer screening age to 45 years, and the heightened recognition of a wide spectrum of syndromic populations that require frequent and close-interval endoscopic surveillance (Lynch syndrome, familial adenomatous polyposis, Peutz-Jeghers syndrome, among others). There already exists a shortage of gastroenterologists in the country, and many communities experience delayed access to endoscopy.[22] Coupled with forces of attrition such as the burden of increasingly complex electronic medical records, physician burnout, decreased reimbursement, and an aging workforce, this increased demand for procedures places an even greater strain on outpatient gastroenterologists.

With Centers for Medicare and Medicaid Services (CMS) formally publishing the Physician Fee Schedule for 2021, declining reimbursements continue to be a threat to GI practices. The calendar year (CY) 2021 Physician Fee Schedule conversion factor is $34.89, representing a decrease of $1.20 from the 2020 conversion factor of $36.09.[23] As such, GI practices must increasingly focus on office schedule efficiency and maximizing patient encounters to offset the per-service reduction in reimbursement. A GI hospitalist model allows outpatient gastroenterologists to avoid disruptions to their outpatient office schedules. In turn, although highly dependent on the characteristics of the patient population as well as the nature of the clinical scenarios encountered, this increased outpatient consultation volume should generate an increase in procedural volume.

The once-traditional model of a gastroenterologist providing concurrent inpatient and outpatient care is becoming less tenable (**Fig. 1**). Outpatient gastroenterologists can no longer afford to cancel office appointments or elective procedures to accommodate inpatient emergencies or allow entire clinical sessions to go unused if relegated to inpatient coverage for set periods of time. The role of the GI hospitalist allows outpatient gastroenterologists to maintain both office appointments and outpatient endoscopy schedules without disruption. It also removes the need for outpatient gastroenterologists to reserve endoscopy time for inpatient procedures, thereby maximizing throughput, endoscopic efficiency, and reimbursement at the AEC. All too often, systems with outpatient gastroenterologists covering inpatient endoscopy find themselves paying staff for overtime or staffing for after-hours availability because of the outpatient gastroenterologist's other responsibilities and schedule. Moving to a GI hospitalist model is cost saving with less need for overtime pay and reduced stress on staff.

Certain GI hospitalist models incorporate some outpatient endoscopy depending on individual interests and practice needs. Practices that employ multiple GI hospitalists may have providers with allocated weeks of out-of-hospital or off-service time. These providers can provide essential coverage for unused endoscopy sessions in HOPDs or AECs when their outpatient colleagues are on vacation or, as seen during the coronavirus disease 2019 (COVID-19) pandemic, can provide sick-coverage if a provider is unexpectedly unable to work. Building this maximization of human resources into the GI practice can help significantly reduce financial losses by avoiding procedure cancelations and improving access to procedures that the practice may otherwise struggle to accommodate.

The benefit of the GI hospitalist model extends to increasing practice visibility, improving relations, and expanding referral networks within the health system. As a stable presence within the hospital, GI hospitalists become an important source for referrals by funneling follow-up visits and procedures to their outpatient colleagues. They also become a reliable and familiar presence that primary teams, emergency room providers, and other consultants can refer to. Significant outpatient procedure

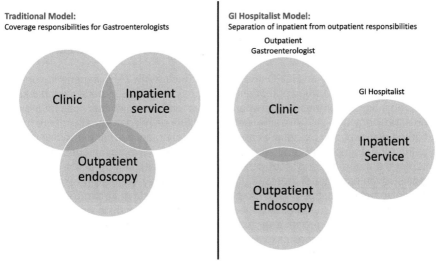

Traditional Model:
Coverage responsibilities for Gastroenterologists

GI Hospitalist Model:
Separation of inpatient from outpatient responsibilities

Fig. 1. Traditional models consisted of gastroenterologists providing concurrent inpatient and outpatient care. The GI hospitalist model allows the outpatient gastroenterologist to maintain office and outpatient endoscopy schedules without disruption.

volumes can be generated from inpatient consultation so it is important to ensure that an efficient system is in place to capture deferred or follow-up procedures by the outpatient practice.

HOSPITAL OUTPATIENT DEPARTMENT

Special consideration needs to be given to hospital-based endoscopy centers where both outpatient and inpatient procedures are performed. As mentioned earlier, GI hospitalists are ever-present in hospital endoscopy units and have a unique perspective on unit efficiency. They can work to improve throughput and maximize efficiency by working on systems improvement initiatives as well as providing a consistent presence to troubleshoot issues that may arise day to day and pose delays in care. In addition, because they are dedicated to inpatient coverage, they are present throughout the day for any urgent or emergent add-on procedures and can quickly accommodate these additional procedures without causing significant disruption to provider schedules. This presence allows the potential for more procedures to be completed on any given day for inpatients and helps alleviate strain on their outpatient colleagues. Overall, using a GI hospitalist model can result in significant increases in endoscopic volume for a practice, whether inpatient or outpatient, HOPD or AEC. Examination of the impact of a GI hospitalist model at 1 center showed an increase in total endoscopic procedures of 20% (P = .01), with 19% (P = .02) in outpatient and 22% (P<.001) in inpatient procedural volume.[24]

A unique benefit inherent to a mixed HOPD endoscopy center is that the GI hospitalists can also be used to support their outpatient colleagues with unanticipated outpatient procedures. For example, if a patient presenting for screening colonoscopy has a poor bowel prep, and the outpatient gastroenterologist has a full office schedule the following day, this patient can be instructed to remain on a clear liquid diet, perform a modified bowel prep, and return to the endoscopy suite for the screening colonoscopy to be completed by the GI hospitalist. In the case of scheduling conflicts, such as misbooked procedures when the outpatient attending is in clinic or on vacation, or the patient shows up unexpectedly, prepped for a colonoscopy that was in fact scheduled for a month later, there is typically enough flexibility in the inpatient endoscopy schedule for the GI hospitalists to perform the outpatient procedures for their colleagues.

GI practices with only an HOPD and no free-standing ASC/AEC experience unique challenges. At the point when outpatient endoscopy schedules experience a backlog, there is an inherent competition between inpatient and outpatient services for the use of the endoscopy unit. At 1 extreme, certain institutions relegate inpatient time to the end of the day or during outpatient cancelations and no-shows. Other models devote an entire room to inpatient procedures. Both scenarios have advantages and disadvantages. Although the endoscopy center that maximizes its outpatient endoscopy schedule at the expense of inpatient procedure time may be more profitable for the outpatient practice, inpatients may experience undue delays in care or suboptimal care if endoscopic procedures are then performed emergently in nonideal settings such as in the operating room after hours. Endoscopy centers that devote an entire room to inpatient procedures risk wasting fixed resources such as nursing and anesthesia staff if the day is light. Further challenges exist in a mixed endoscopy center with anesthesia staff that may be untrained or uncomfortable in managing higher-risk American Society of Anesthesiologists (ASA) Physical Status Classification System III and IV patients with multiple comorbidities and variable clinical stability. As such, it is important to design endoscopy schedules at an HOPD that match the average demand for inpatient procedures, and to select anesthesia staff capable of and willing to care for higher-risk inpatients.

ROLE OF THE GASTROENTEROLOGY HOSPITALIST IN ADVANCED ENDOSCOPY

Dr Kathy Bull-Henry details opportunities for GI hospitalists in advanced therapeutic endoscopy in Video 5.

Advances in technology including endoscopic ultrasonography, endoscopic retrograde cholangiopancreatography, and single-balloon and double-balloon enteroscopy have greatly increased the spectrum of diagnostic and therapeutic services that can be offered by advanced endoscopists. The traditional model for managing patients in need of advanced endoscopy consists of an advanced therapeutic endoscopy team separate from the general GI service. This team is led by a therapeutic GI attending who sees the initial consult, performs the therapeutic procedure, and coordinates all preprocedure and postprocedure care. However, in this model, advanced endoscopists typically have busy outpatient practices with backlogs of outpatient endoscopic procedures, particularly if they practice at tertiary care referral centers. Given the highly specialized nature of these procedures, the advanced endoscopy attendings' schedules are greatly affected by any duties that detract from their endoscopy time. Days or weeks on call performing general inpatient GI service can translate to a significant increase in wait times for outpatients in need of advanced procedures. The GI hospitalist model as described previously would allow the on-call advanced therapeutic gastroenterologists to maintain much of their outpatient endoscopy schedules while being available for inpatient advanced procedures. This model works particularly well in the HOPD.

In order to maximize the advanced endoscopists' time spent performing procedures, some practices have turned to hiring an APP to perform inpatient consults and follow-up care for hospitalized patients in need of advanced GI care. In this model, the advanced attending is able to remain in the endoscopy unit performing advanced procedures. However, the training involved to produce a capable independent APP for advanced GI services is likely to take a significant amount of time and effort. Other practices have recruited general GI hospitalists to manage the initial consultations, follow-ups, and coordination of care for both general GI and advanced therapeutic patients. In some settings, the GI hospitalists are trained in various therapeutic procedures such as deep enteroscopy and luminal stenting, based on their interest, skill, and comfort level. In addition, some institutions have employed GI hospitalists with advanced endoscopy training. The success of such a model depends highly on the inpatient volume of consults and procedures, as well as on the ability and interest level of the GI hospitalist to manage both general and advanced cases.

In light of this model where the GI hospitalist can perform both general and advanced endoscopy, there is a growing opportunity for interventional endoscopy–trained fellows to explore careers as GI hospitalists. Particularly in areas with a high volume of outpatient gastroenterologists performing advanced procedures, advanced endoscopy fellows fresh out of training are more likely to maintain and expand their skills if they can become hospitalists focusing on advanced procedures. However, this model may lead to some outpatient physicians gaining experience with endoscopic retrograde cholangiopancreatography (ERCP) only when on call. When time-consuming procedures such as endoscopic mucosal resection, endoscopic submucosal dissection, and deep enteroscopy are commonly part of the GI hospitalist's day, it becomes even more important that someone else, be it a general GI hospitalist, an APP, or an advanced GI fellow, is able to provide coverage for inpatient consults and care coordination.

FUTURE DIRECTIONS: QUALITY AND VALUE-BASED CARE

Dr Glenn Littenberg describes future directions for the GI hospitalist model in Video 6, particularly in quality measurement and in the transition from fee-for-service to value-based care.

Thus far, the discussion has revolved around how the GI hospitalist model improves endoscopic efficiency, throughput, and patient access to procedures (**Fig. 2**). Highlighted next is how GI hospitalists have the potential to play an integral role in quality measurement and monitoring, and in helping practices transition from fee-for-service to value-based care models.

For inpatient endoscopy, studying the proportion of canceled procedures and their causes (poor bowel prep, clinical instability, lack of cardiac or anesthesia clearance) can provide great insight for optimizing inpatient procedures. The GI hospitalists are naturally the most invested and appropriate practice members to oversee these investigations. Given their knowledge of the hospital system's pain points, GI hospitalists are also best positioned to lead hospital-based quality improvement and patient safety initiatives. Further studies are warranted in examining the conditions that allow the GI hospitalist model to improve patient satisfaction while reducing hospital length of stay, redundant procedures, readmissions, cost of care, and mortality.[25]

Other quality metrics, such as those related to endoscopy, are a main focus for both practices and payors. Although certain areas of medicine are further along in the evolution toward value-based care in all aspects of practice, endoscopy remains rooted largely in fee-for-service models. GI hospitalists are more likely to follow standard of care for management of disorders (such as bleeding peptic ulcers) that may be unfamiliar to providers who only rotate for a few weeks every year on the inpatient service. They are also more likely to provide thorough documentation and coding that more

Endoscopic Practice Area	Potential Impact of the GI Hospitalist
Inpatient Endoscopy	Efficiency with managing acute care
	Improved time from consult to inpatient endoscopy
	Reduced length of stay
	Improved collaboration with ancillary services
	Greater inpatient service continuity
	Potential for increased quality of care and greater opportunities for quality initiatives and monitoring
Outpatient Endoscopy (AEC or ASC)	Decreased disruptions to outpatient schedules
	Improved access for screening/surveillance and diagnostic endoscopic procedures
Hospital-based Outpatient Endoscopy	Improved throughput and efficiency
	Increased flexibility and accommodation for emergent add-on procedures

Fig. 2. The GI hospitalist model has the potential to benefit inpatient endoscopy and outpatient endoscopy through greater efficiency in managing acute care, decreased disruptions to outpatient schedules, and improving patient access to endoscopic procedures.

accurately reflect patient risk of mortality and severity of illness, which affects billing for both the practice and the health system.

When a hospitalized patient is stable for discharge but warrants an endoscopic procedure, the GI hospitalist can shift the hospital procedure to be performed by an outpatient colleague at the practice's AEC. This assured near-term outpatient procedure results in a shortened hospital length of stay and thus a decrease in health care use and cost. GI hospitalists play a significant role in selecting the setting in which endoscopic procedures are performed and in eliminating unnecessary procedures when medical management is indicated.

Hospitalized patients in need for more urgent outpatient follow-up can be scheduled within 1-week or 2-week time frames to allow for transitional care management (TCM). These clinics can also improve interdepartmental relationships with other specialists, emergency departments, and primary care providers. The GI practice benefits from the associated enhanced TCM reimbursement. Payors and hospitals benefit from the resultant reduction in readmissions or emergency room encounters. To support these clinics, APPs or other provider staffing may be required. In some hospitalist models, where multiple GI hospitalists are used within a practice, GI hospitalists themselves may staff half-day or full-day TCM clinic sessions during the weeks they are not on inpatient service.

However, it is important that GI hospitalist compensation structures align with the goals of the practice and institution. In a purely fee-for-service model, GI hospitalist salaries based solely on work relative value units (RVUs) and productivity may lead to procedures being performed in the hospital that would be more appropriate for the AEC, or might be only marginally indicated. Furthermore, GI hospitalists have little control over consultation or procedure volume and payor mix. As such, salaries based solely on work RVUs and net collections may unfairly penalize the GI hospitalists when productivity is lower than expected, for factors largely beyond their control. A proposed compensation structure consists of a base salary for full-time GI hospitalist physicians with a work RVU threshold in line with GI inpatient standards. Cross-subsidization arrangements from the GI practice or from the hospital toward the GI hospitalist's salary may be necessary. Compensation structures may even incorporate incentives based on such outcomes as hospital length of stay, patient satisfaction, timeliness of consultation, time to endoscopy, and success of transitions of care.

SUMMARY

Modern GI practice has benefited from tremendous enhancements in clinical care algorithms and technology in relation to patients with GI illness and in the realm of endoscopic practice. In addition, several new paradigms have emerged under the auspices of the Affordable Care Act, with a renewed emphasis on quality of care, patient satisfaction, and improving outcomes. More value and higher quality are expected despite decreasing reimbursements and higher costs of practice. Given these trends, optimizing endoscopic operations must revolve around improving efficiency, patient access to procedures, and quality of care.

As detailed in this article, the use of GI hospitalists provides the opportunity to improve coordination of care for hospitalized patients, while increasing endoscopic efficiency and referrals for their outpatient colleagues. Inpatient GI care stands to benefit from this paradigm with improved communication, multidisciplinary care coordination, and access to more timely high-quality care. Outpatient gastroenterologists experience fewer disruptions to both their office and outpatient endoscopy schedules, resulting in greater endoscopy unit use, efficiency, and profitability.

Future directions for the GI hospitalist model involve exploring more ways to leverage this paradigm. Key areas moving forward will include expanding the role of GI hospitalists and the teams that supports them, using advanced endoscopists as GI hospitalists, and developing compensation strategies that more fairly and accurately account for the work and value the GI hospitalists bring to practices and to hospitals. Although the impetus for the GI hospital model revolves around high-quality patient-centered inpatient care, the benefits of this paradigm are far-reaching and work in many ways to optimize endoscopic operations for the entire GI practice.

CLINICS CARE POINTS

- GI hospitalists gain expertise in managing critically ill patients and endoscopic emergencies, which can translate into increased efficiency for the inpatient endoscopy unit.

- GI hospitalists are ideally positioned to meet increasing demands for GI specialty consultation for the increasingly high case index (severity, age) of GI inpatients, including, for example, the growing population of patients at risk for gastrointestinal bleeding from newer anticoagulants.

- Outpatient gastroenterologists benefit from the GI hospitalist model with increased efficiency in their office appointments and outpatient endoscopy schedules.

- Value-based care arrangements benefit from the efficiency of GI hospitalists to triage less serious patients, or procedures that can be deferred or replaced by medical management, to the outpatient environment more expeditiously.

- New models of GI hospitalist compensation structures should consider cross-subsidization from revenue generated at the ASC and the hospital while incorporating outcome-based incentives that align with the goals of the practice and the hospital.

DISCLOSURE

The authors have nothing relevant to disclose.

SUPPLEMENTARY DATA

Supplementary data related to this article can be found online at https://doi.org/10.1016/j.giec.2021.05.005.

REFERENCES

1. Wachter RM, Goldman L. Zero to 50,000 - The 20th Anniversary of the Hospitalist. N Engl J Med 2016;375(11):1009–11.
2. Wachter RM, Goldman L. The Emerging role of "Hospitalists" in the American Health Care System. N Engl J Med 1996;335(7):514–7.
3. Klein JP. The Academic Neurohospitalist: Building a Successful Career and Practice. Ann Neurol 2015;78(4):515–9.
4. Gorelick PB, Schneck MJ, Glisson C. A new era of neurologic practice, the need to shift the residency training paradigm, and the importance of hospitalist neurology. Neurohospitalist 2013;3(3):117–9.
5. Messler J, Whitcomb WF. A History of the Hospitalist Movement. Obstet Gynecol Clin North Am 2015;42(3):419–32.
6. Hughes M, Sun E, Enslin S, et al. The role of the gastroenterology hospitalist in modern practice. Gastroenterol Hepatol 2020;16(11):571–6.
7. Allen JI, Aldrich L, Moote M. Building a team-based gastroenterology practice with advanced practice providers. Gastroenterol Hepatol 2019;15(4):213–20.
8. Allen J, Hutchinson A, Brown R, et al. Quality care outcomes following transitional care interventions for older people from hospital to home: a systematic review. BMC Health Serv Res 2014;14:346.
9. Cai Q, Bruno CJ, Hagedorn CH, et al. Temporal trends over ten years in formal inpatient gastroenterology consultation at an inner-city hospital. J Clin Gastroenterol 2003;36(1):34–8.
10. Bohra S, Byrne MF, Manning D, et al. A prospective analysis of inpatient consultation to a gastroenterology service. Ir Med J 2003;96(9):263–5.
11. Pines JM, Mullins PM, Cooper JK, et al. National trends in emergency department use, care patterns, and quality of care of older adults in the United States. J Am Geriatr Soc 2013;61(1):12–7.
12. Sun R, Karaca Z, Wong H. Trends in hospital emergency department visits by age and payer, 2006-2015. HCUP statistical Brief #238. Rockville (MD): Agency for Healthcare Research and Quality; 2018. Available at: https://www.hcup-us.ahrq.gov/reports/statbriefs/sb238-Emergency-Department-Age-Payer-2006-2015.pdf. Accessed December 20, 2020.
13. Are Medicare Patients Getting Sicker? In: American Hospital Association TRENDWATCH. 2012. Available at: https://www.aha.org/system/files/2018-06/2012-are-medicare-pts-getting-sicker-trendwatch.pdf. Accessed December 20, 2020.
14. Lanas A, García-Rodríguez LA, Polo-Tomás M, et al. Time trends and impact of upper and lower gastrointestinal bleeding and perforation in clinical practice. Am J Gastroenterol 2009;104(7):1633–41.
15. Sorensen R, Hansen ML, Abildstrom SZ, et al. Risk of bleeding in patients with acute myocardial infarction treated with different combinations of aspirin, clopidogrel, and vitamin K antagonists in Denmark: a retrospective analysis of nationwide registry data. Lancet 2009;374(9706):1967–74.

16. Mahadev S, Lebwohl B, Ramirez I, et al. Mo1115: Transition to a GI hospitalist system is associated with expedited upper endoscopy. Gastroenterology 2016; 150(4):S639–40.
17. Maa J, Carter JT, Gosnell JE, et al. The surgical hospitalist: a new model for emergency surgical care. J Am Coll Surg 2007;205(5):704–11.
18. Srinivas SK, Small DS, Macheras M, et al. Evaluating the impact of the laborist model on obstetric care on maternal and neonatal outcomes. Am J Obstet Gynecol 2016;215(6):770.e1-9.
19. Ireye BK, Huang WH, Condon J, et al. Implementation of a laborist program and evaluation of the effect upon cesarean delivery. Am J Obstet Gynecol 2013; 209(3):251e1–6.
20. Schoeppner HL, Miller SL. Developing a gastroenterology hospitalist service. Gastrointest Endosc Clin N Am 2006;16(4):743–50.
21. Yang D, Summerlee R, Suarez A, et al. Evaluation of interventional endoscopy unit efficiency metrics at a tertiary academic medical center. Endosc Int Open 2016;04:E143–8.
22. Pallardy C. What gastroenterologists can expect from a physician shortage. In Becker's GI & Endoscopy. 2015. Available at: https://www.beckersasc.com/gastroenterology-and-endoscopy/what-gastroenterologists-can-expect-from-a-physician-shortage.html. Accessed December 20, 2020.
23. Physician Fee Schedule. CY 2021 Physician Fee Schedule Update. 2021. Available at: https://www.cms.gov/Medicare/Medicare-Fee-for-Service-Payment/PhysicianFeeSched. Accessed January 14, 2021.
24. Shung D, Hung K, Laine L, et al. Adopting a GI hospitalist model: a new method for increasing procedural volume. Am J Gastroenterol 2020;115:s259.
25. Wray CM, Flores A, Padula WV, et al. Measuring patient experiences on hospitalist and teaching services: patient responses to a 30-day postdischarge questionnaire. J Hosp Med 2016;11(2):99–104.

Navigating and Leveraging Social Media

Austin L. Chiang, MD, MPH[a,b,c,]*

KEYWORDS

- Social media • Gastroenterology • Health education • Information dissemination
- Marketing of health services • Online social networking • Organizational policy

KEY POINTS

- Social media plays a pivotal role in dissemination of health information.
- Various social medial platforms exist, serving different groups of audiences.
- Medical misinformation remains a substantial challenge for health care professional to navigate.

INTRODUCTION

Social media has shaped how we communicate with one another across various sectors, including health care. One example of the tremendous influence social media has on public health has been the Coronavirus Disease 2019 (COVID-19) pandemic. However, despite this impact, learning how to navigate and leverage social media is not included in a standard medical school curriculum. This article aims to fill the gaps in understanding how to navigate and leverage social media as a clinician.

Social media is most often described as Web 2.0 internet-based applications that facilitate online interaction often through user-generated content shared within a social network.[1] Today, 4.2 billion people or 53% of the global population is estimated to be on social media.[2] On average, individuals spend over 2 hours per day on social media. Whether actively searching for information on social media or passively consuming social media, social media can potentially impact public health through influencing public opinion.

Over the years, there has been a growing presence of health professionals using social media in a multitude of ways across various social media platforms. Developing an online presence is not always intuitive, and getting started on social media requires an evaluation of one's communication strengths, purpose for being online, and an understanding of which platform would be most suitable. Even after attracting an audience through consistent engagement over time, there are also potential pitfalls to heed.

[a] Sidney Kimmel Medical College; [b] Endoscopic Bariatric Program, Thomas Jefferson University Hospital; [c] Jefferson Health
* Thomas Jefferson University Hospital, 132 South 10th Street, Philadelphia, PA 19107, USA
E-mail address: austin.chiang@jefferson.edu

Gastrointest Endoscopy Clin N Am 31 (2021) 695–707
https://doi.org/10.1016/j.giec.2021.05.006
1052-5157/21/© 2021 Elsevier Inc. All rights reserved.

Practitioners, professional organizations, medical journals, and patients in gastro-enterology (GI) have been present on various social media platforms in varying capacities depending on their goals and interests. Compared to other fields, gastroenterologists' adoption of social media in general has lagged behind other medical subspecialties. Up to 62% of patients with inflammatory bowel disease expressed interest in learning from their gastroenterologists on social media.[3–5] Social media platforms have allowed gastroenterologists to not only network but also disseminate health information that could potentially directly impact public health or indirectly influence clinical practice. A recent Twitter poll, for instance, helped elucidate differences in interpreting urgency of procedures within the context of the COVID-19 pandemic.[6]

It may also be that different patient groups seek health information on different platforms. However, when it comes to gastroenterological information online, misinformation abounds. One study found that the number of videos incompletely describing bowel preparation outnumbered those that were more comprehensive in their descriptions.[7] Another found that the quality of YouTube videos about gastroesophageal reflux disease was low.[8] Although some patients are already skeptical of health information on the internet, physicians should better understand what is being presented to patients on social media and how to potentially use social media to bolster accurate information.

SOCIAL MEDIA PLATFORMS

Although not limited to mobile devices, social media is often associated with specific mobile applications (apps) that run these social media platforms. Among the largest social media applications are Facebook, Instagram, Twitter, YouTube, LinkedIn, and TikTok.

Twitter

Launched in March 2006, Twitter is a microblogging platform that allows users to share posts or "tweets" limited to 280 characters or less. Since its inception, Twitter has evolved also several different built-in features such as polling functions, quote tweets, and Fleets—the latest addition of 24-hour time-limited photo or video highlights following the success of Snapchat and Instagram stories. Twitter's explore page within the app also features a ranked list of trending phrases or topics that reflects the real-time zeitgeist.

Currently, Twitter boasts 353 million active users.[9] Twitter is often regarded as the most popular social media platform among academic physicians, including both trainees and faculty members. Here you can expect individuals engaging freeform academic discussion as well as regularly scheduled chats. Medical professionals on social media use Twitter not only to communicate with one another but also to promote public health messaging and educate patients as their intended audience. Yet other individual accounts have also used the platform to advocate for personal interests or causes affecting patient care. By "tagging" other individuals or groups within one's tweet, ideas promulgated through Twitter can at times garner widespread, "viral" attention and ignite further media coverage and interest. Although Twitter once displayed tweets in chronologic order, nowadays tweets are presented according to an algorithm that predicts content of most interest to the user. Before the search function, clicking into hashtags (phrases preceded by "#") were the only way to access content relevant to your own interests. Today, hashtags serve to assist the algorithm in identifying similar topics. In 2016, major GI journals and societies present on the app were assembled to create a standardized list of hashtags to better curate academic discussion.[10]

Not only are there thought leaders and social media influencers within the professional community, but all major gastroenterological societies and journals maintain active Twitter presences. GI societies have been able to quickly disseminate organizational updates, promote society events and courses, and engage their membership. Likewise, journals can rapidly promote newly accepted publications far ahead of print versions. This has been particularly important during the COVID-19 pandemic where timely release of new information was critical.

Facebook

Founded in 2004, Facebook is the largest social media network with over 2.74 billion monthly active users.[11] Originally a networking site, Facebook has blossomed into a complex platform that serves groups, professional/business pages, a marketplace, a video platform, and a messaging app among other features. As the largest social platform, Facebook promises the visibility advertisers seek. Although not entirely an original concept, the main content feed with its constant stream of posts, photos, and videos has set the stage for other social media platforms that came after.

For gastroenterologists, perhaps the most important and distinguishing feature about Facebook is groups where patients and professionals can congregate around specific interests. One study showed that professional engagement with patient groups may be an effective way of providing women with colorectal cancer risk reduction information.[12] In addition, Facebook's advertising reach should be considered for not only practice marketing but also for the potential impact advertised products (especially those that may carry health risk) may have on our patients.

Instagram

Instagram was introduced in 2010 and bought by Facebook in 2012 for $1 billion. It commands 1 billion monthly users and 140 million American users.[13] Similar to Facebook and other social media platforms, the original concept was rather simple but then became increasingly complex over time with the introduction of many features and parallel content feeds. The original concept consisted of a main feed that features images (and more recently videos) paired with captions posted by those who are followed by the user. Content was previously presented in chronologic order, but an algorithm was later introduced to predict content in order of interest. The captions allow users to expound more extensively than Twitter with a character limit up to 2200 characters. Since 2013, Instagram has also incorporated direct messaging ("DM") capabilities within the app between users or groups of users. In 2016, Instagram Stories was introduced, where users can post time-limited photos or videos that expire after 24 hours, with the ability to add certain features such as question and answer fields, polling function, stickers, music, and the ability to swipe to view external links (generally available to those with over 10,000 followers). In 2018, IGTV was introduced to house long-form video content at least 1 minute in duration. In 2020, the platform introduced Reels, which can be described as a competitor of Tik-Tok in the way that it is short-form video (up to 30 seconds in duration) presented in a separate feed to those who are not following the user. Similar to Twitter, Instagram users often use hashtags to help the application curate content and present posts to those interested in similar content.

At the moment, there are a handful of gastroenterologists on Instagram, some of whom are trainees and others who are practicing in both academia or in private practice. Given the relevant scarcity of gastroenterologists on Instagram, the community is relatively tight knit and not siloed by specialty as noticeably as on Twitter.

YouTube

YouTube is a video-based social media platform first launched in 2005. Boasting over 2 billion active monthly users, YouTube also is considered the second largest search engine in the world after Google, with whom it shares a parent company (Alphabet Inc). From an individual clinician perspective, barrier to entry is high given the required understanding of video production experience and the time often required to produce and edit video content. However, the platform is unique in its searchability, and it has a mature model for monetizing video-related content. More than 500 hours of video content are uploaded every minute (or roughly 82 years worth of video content everyday). Similar to many other social media platforms, YouTube has also adopted many other functionalities such as image- or text-based community social media posts, live-streaming, and YouTube Shorts—short-form video and the platform's latest addition that lives evergreen on the platform, unlike Instagram stories or Snapchat snaps.

TikTok

TikTok was derived from Chinese equivalent Douyin and introduced outside of China in 2017. In 2018, the platform merged with Musical.ly. As of July 2020, it was described as the fastest growing social media network of all time with 2 billion downloads and 100 million monthly active users in the United States. The platform consists of the main feed or "For You" page, which possesses a format and algorithm where content has the potential to reach anyone's "For You" page (and not just those who follow the creator or are associated with the creator in some fashion). The "For You" page features the most engaging, "viral" content. Since late 2019, there has been a surge in health professionals joining the platform, but still very few gastroenterologists. Some health professionals express hesitancy in joining the platform, as TikTok content is video form only, and is often set to music, dancing, or humor to attract viewership. Because of its often comedic format, several health professional creators have been publicly criticized or disciplined for content deemed controversial or unprofessional.[14] However, the incredible reach of the platform has also seen productive use in promoting evidence-based, educational content centered around subspecialty topics or general public health concepts such as vaccine awareness.[15,16]

Other Platforms

It is important to note that the transmission of health-related content is not limited to the aforementioned platforms. Apart from traditional media outlets, many popular other social media platforms have also seen considerable popularity such as Snapchat, Reddit, Pinterest, and more recently Clubhouse. These platforms may also foster health-related discussions and be at risk for health misinformation or disinformation. Although sometimes overlooked as social media applications, other messaging platforms such as WhatsApp, WeChat, Line, or Discord may also be contributing to the propagation of health misinformation as well.

LEVERAGING SOCIAL MEDIA

Many mistakenly believe that audiences will naturally flock to social media content, achieving virality with ease. But exposure on social media is inconsistent, as platforms have moved away from a chronologic display of content and are now using algorithms to predict and cater to the interests of their users. In other words, because social media platforms are also trying to retain the attention of their users, exposure on social media is subject to the whims of platform algorithms to determine whether content will show up at the top of one's feed, lower in the feed, or not at all. While algorithms cannot be altered, optimizing other elements such as one's social media identity or the content itself can be cultivated to improve the odds of exposure.

Group accounts often attract less of a following than individual accounts. This also varies by platform, as medical journals and organizations have still been able to build sizable followings. There are also some data to suggest an association between social media activity by medical journals and manuscript citations.[17] But regardless of an individual or group presence, social media exposure is also dependent on numerous metrics including one's existing following, the extent to which they are interested and engaged with your content, how long they remain on a piece of content ("watch time"), whether they watch videos or click through to other elements embedded in your content, or how many "likes", "comments", or "shares" the video garners. Augmenting one's engagement also involves developing brand recognition. This can be achieved in part through consistent conceptual and visual messaging across platforms and consistent engagement with one's audience. Catering content to one's existing audience can be improved through review of one's social media analytics. Most established social media platforms provide various degrees of insight into one's audience demographics and viewing/engagement patterns. Another method to broaden one's reach and attract followers or subscribers would be to collaborate with like-minded creators, which simultaneously facilitates integration into the online community. Social media collaborations often appear in multiple formats including interviews, guest appearances, or larger awareness campaigns. These campaigns are often anchored around a particular hashtag, which curates all content surrounding the hashtag for interested audiences and promotes content around the hashtag to the feeds of others.

IDENTIFYING PURPOSE

In a deluge of social media posts, producing content that is novel, thought-provoking, and "on brand" can be challenging. Leveraging social media is nuanced and involves a calculated approach toward one's online purpose, target audience, platform selection, individual strengths, and personal interests among other factors. There is no single permutation of the aforementioned factors that guarantees "success," given frequent changes in public interest and the social platforms themselves. Ideally, the platform structure is also aligned with one's own strengths in communication, whether in format (such as text, photographs, illustrations, short-form or long-form video) or expression (such as didactic, humorous, or artistic forms).

The initial step is identifying one's purpose on social media, which will then determine the target audience and most suitable social media platform to select as a launching point. At times a social media presence can serve more than one purpose, and none are mutually exclusive. Although certain goals such as combating misinformation may be a byproduct of another primary purpose (such as interprofessional education), exploring different motivations in social media may inform the ideal approach.

Patient Education and Dispelling Misinformation

In 2013, the Pew Internet Project study reported 72% of internet users search online for health information.[18] However, a potentially greater percentage of individuals are exposed to health information on the internet even without actively searching for it.

Unfortunately, trust in the medical profession has declined from 73% in 1966 to 34% in 2012.[19] Although 58% agreed that doctors could be trusted in the United States, this percentage was 24th among 29 industrialized countries (with Switzerland ranking first at 83%).[19] Addressing this mistrust, in part, requires physicians and health professionals to be present and visible on social media platforms where health information is consumed. Educating patients directly or indirectly through online discourse may help restore trust in health care, improve health literacy, and improve clinical outcomes. There is also potential for direct use of social media as an adjunct to a treatment plan. For instance, patients who received reminders delivered through social media platforms seemed to demonstrate improved knowledge and adherence to *Helicobacter pylori* treatment compared with the control group.[20]

Trust in the medical profession is lacking, in part due to rampant medical misinformation and disinformation on the internet. Specific to GI, there are numerous accounts across social media platforms promoting non–evidence-based gut health tips as well as supplements, home remedies and treatment methods of constipation, and other strategies for gut or liver "detoxification", cancer prevention, and weight loss.[21] Even popular topics such as colonoscopy are plagued by an abundance of low-quality videos on YouTube.[22] Content from multiple social media platforms appears to promote self-administered fecal microbiota transplantation (FMT) or inappropriate indications for FMT.[23] Establishing a social media presence allows appropriately credentialed professionals to proactively spread accurate information or respond to erroneous content.

However, nonprofessional accounts are not all to blame. At times, the brevity of social media content may be prone to deficiencies in detail or context. Other times, even with reputable sources, results may be misinterpreted or presented incorrectly. One study investigated a sample of academic studies shared on social media, noting there were high rates of causal inference despite 70% lacking strength of inference and that 58% inaccurately reported questions, results, intervention, or population of the study.[24]

Elevating Recognition of Gastroenterology

Certain subspecialty areas within GI such as advanced endoscopy or transplant hepatology may be less recognized and understood by members of the general public. Addressing misperceptions about GI may help patients and the general public better understand the multiple roles gastroenterologists serve within health care. Awareness of these areas may be lacking because some of the associated diseases and conditions are less publicized or receive less marketing funding than others. Introducing these fields to the general public could also potentially inspire aspiring physicians and attract younger audiences to the field. A greater health professional presence online may also help in providing professional responses to timely events such as medical breakthroughs or celebrity diagnoses relevant to GI conditions.

Gastroenterologists who educate on social media may also attract patients seeking care within their communities. Patient engagement with their own physicians on social media may help build loyalty and prevent attrition. Where relevant, physicians can also leverage social media to recruit patients for clinical trials, develop other business endeavors such as consulting opportunities, and launch other community initiatives.

An active social media presence by individual physicians or group accounts may help improve institutional ranking via greater promotion of a division or practice's achievements and greater recognition by the local or national GI community as a result. One study found that institutional follower count on Twitter was an independent predictor of divisional ranking and reputation score as defined by U.S. News and World Report and that an institutional increase in 8000 followers predicted a maintained or higher divisional rank after 2 years.[25]

Humanizing Medicine and Self Expression

Social media provides yet another method that patients can communicate with physicians and an extra layer of understanding to relate to those who diagnose and treat them. Patients may empathize with physicians and their triumphs, struggles, interests, and ideals. Depending on the platform and audience, health professionals have showcased facets of their personality (through humor, dance, commentary) alongside their professional journey as a counterpoint to the perception that doctors are intimidating and unapproachable. These platforms also allow patients to follow and potentially communicate with their practitioners either in publicly visible comment sections or in direct one-on-one messaging. This, however, must be approached gingerly within the guardrails of ethical conduct and professionalism.

Social media is often used as an outlet for self-expression, and health professionals are able to connect with others outside of the field to cultivate other interests. Even from a professional perspective, there is opportunity for collaboration and discussion across disciplines that may lead to new areas of study within medicine. Known for his artistic interpretations of clinical scenarios, Dr Michael Natter was featured in a series titled "Annals Graphic Medicine" in the *Annals of Internal Medicine*.[26,27]

Professional Education and Networking

Social media has allowed gastroenterologists to connect with others within the specialty and externally outside the specialty across various platforms. For trainees, the access to leaders, division leadership, and other leaders in the field is greater than ever before. Social media connection may also foster community among different subspecialties and groups within GI, especially through participation in structured chats around specialized topics.

The concept of free open-access online medical education (FOAMed) is a movement founded in 2012 curated under the hashtag #FOAMed, originally focused on emergency medicine and critical care topics.[28] More recently, unstructured conversations in FOAMed have been centered around the COVID-19 pandemic.[29] Multiple structured, educational chats are hosted by specific accounts (eg, @MondayNight-IBD, @GIJournalClub, @ScopingSundays) on Twitter with content curated under their respective hashtags #MondayNightIBD, #GIJC, and #ScopingSundays. #MondayNightIBD's CME-accreditation further reflects the bona fide role Twitter serves as an educational platform. Another common format for education on Twitter is the "Tweetorial" where a string of tweets is presented in success to depict a concept or to discuss a medical publication. "Live tweeting" courses and conference has also been a method of providing educational value between colleagues, who at times may not be able to attend these events. The perception of social media use among GI fellowship program directors has also shifted over the years. There has been a significant increase in support for the incorporation of social media into training curricula from 16.9% in 2016 to 35.1% in 2019 ($P = .049$).[30]

The impact of social media on the GI community, on professional development, and on patient understanding and/or clinical outcomes remains largely unknown. Therefore, social media is an opportunity for further study to better understand how gastroenterologists and allied professionals can optimize social media for professional development and public health.

Raising Awareness and Advocacy

The reach of social media may not only help raise awareness about certain causes but also allows professionals from across regions to organize to achieve that goal. Online discourse can potentially yield key insights into challenges that health professionals feel strongly about and could organize around.[31] Although sporadic health messages have the potential to go viral, coordinated social media campaigns with multiple individuals using the same hashtag has a greater likelihood of being noticed by the general public, relevant authority figures, and conventional media. An investigation of the #ThisIsOurLane hashtag with regard to gun violence and #GetUsPPE during the COVID-19 pandemic both appeared to garner more positive, actionable messaging than their nonmedical hashtag counterparts.[32]

NAVIGATING PITFALLS

Although social media is carried out on virtual platforms, its role as an extension of interpersonal interactions and real life is often overlooked. From a physician's perspective, this can be worrisome as it could impact physician-patient relationships and ultimately trust in the health workers at large and public health. With every new social media platform or feature introduced, there are often highly publicized examples of misuse that highlight the pitfalls of professional social media use. The consequences of these missteps can be detrimental to one's career or public image. Fortunately, these occurrences are relatively uncommon and often intuitive to most users. Therefore, the aim of this discussion around pitfalls is to encourage mindful use of social media as a professional, rather than deterring entry into the social media universe.

Before engaging on social media, it is important to review employer and/or institutional social media policies as they can vary widely, at times strictly prohibiting social media use altogether, in a professional capacity, when representing an employer, or solely on hospital property or during work hours. These regulations might vary by practice setting as well, for example, special considerations related to trainee interactions or product endorsements for academic physicians.

At the center of any social media effort is the patient. One of the central tenets to the practice of medicine is protecting patient privacy as outlined by the Health Insurance Portability and Accountability Act (HIPAA). While HIPAA explicitly lists 18 patient identifiers, some of which are self-evident such as name and birth date, other descriptions or images of the patient may inadvertently reveal a patient's identity. Even in the description of patient scenarios, patients and their family members may take offense to public discussion about their care without explicit consent. One study reported family members being able to identify clinical scenarios nearly a third of the time.[33] Radiographs or other procedural images may also reveal jewelry or other unique anatomic features that may reveal patient identity.

A professional online presence often attracts solicitations of personal medical advice. Multiple professional entities and organizations have advised against providing personal medical advice, especially to those who are not under one's care. There is a subtle but clear distinction between questions and answers posed in the context of medical education, as opposed to a personal medical inquiry, where suggestions of intervention may render professionals liable for clinical consequences. It is also important to emphasize that any communication via social media even in private or direct messaging should not be considered confidential. Electronic photo-documentation of these conversations can potentially be published and amplified online.

Preserving the integrity of medical information online is also more challenging than simply reiterating findings from a study. In attempts at debunking misinformation, there is also a risk for further amplifying misinformation as known as the Streisand effect. Similarly, distilling complex medical concepts into bite-sized tweets or 15-second short-form video is sometimes done at the expense of full clinical context and overgeneralization. Citing reputable sources and encouraging followers to refer to primary sources when evaluating online medical content may help mitigate shortcomings of health education on social media.

The risk of perpetuating distrust among the public is ubiquitous in social media. There have been examples of physicians and other professionals acting overtly unprofessional, ranging from mocking patients to expressing discriminatory beliefs. Other times, certain actions or remarks could be considered microaggressions or perpetuating stigma toward certain groups of patients. Furthermore, practitioners must also be mindful of divulging personal information (such as a fatigue or illness) that could be perceived as a potentially affecting clinical performance. Expressing views around polarizing topics or political matters is often up to the discretion of the professional although some employer policies may state otherwise. While some practitioners disclose political stances to advocate in favor of certain health policies or even other nonmedical agendas, others refrain from doing so out of concern that the physician-patient relationship could potentially be affected.

Similarly, a strong social media presence may be followed by concerns about personal safety, online harassment, and intellectual property concerns. A recent study demonstrated that of 464 physicians surveyed, 23.3% reported online harassment, with female physicians more likely to report online sexual harassment (16.4% vs 1.5%, $P<.001$). Other reported instances of harassment included online death threats, stalking, and doxxing (contacting one's employer, fake online reviews). There have also been anecdotal reports of identity theft where physician photographs from social media were used as part of fraudulent activity (eg, phishing scams) or used to promote certain agendas or products without permission. Certain organizations have warned of increased fraud as a result of the COVID-19 pandemic and the increased use of telehealth.

Over the years, the rise of the influencer has also resulted in a cohort of health professionals lending their likeness and professional identity to promote certain products. While regulations about product endorsement vary widely, the Federal Trade Commission outlines specific guidelines for disclosing sponsored content on social media to promote transparency. Guidance specific to medical professionals and industry relationships remains lacking. Although the Sunshine Act was enacted in 2010 to increase transparency between the pharmaceutical or device industry and health professionals, there remains no oversight or enforcement of disclosures of industry conflicts of interest when discussing particular pharmaceuticals, devices, or other therapeutics.

Finally, the time commitment of managing social media accounts and the effects of social media on mental health cannot be ignored. The time and energy devoted to social media should be carefully considered when deciding whether to communicate on multiple platforms. While negative psychological effects of social media have been reported in adolescents and younger individuals, perhaps a similar phenomenon could occur in adults especially when social media platforms invite comparisons with colleagues and display vanity metrics such as followers and "likes." However, others argue in favor of social media as a vehicle to improve mental health of health professionals through finding supportive communities.

Social Media and the Future

Health care social media has garnered greater attention as a result of the COVID-19 pandemic in many ways. It appears that social media platforms have taken note of the impact social media has on public health. For instance, studies have suggested an association between former President Trump's tweets and shifts in public sentiment about the legitimacy and severity of the pandemic.[34] First, social media platforms have looked to health professionals to promote accurate health information. YouTube Health is an initiative to empower more health professionals to put forth evidence-based health information in their areas of expertise. Twitter rushed to provide verification badges to health professionals on its platform to help the general public better identify credible sources of health knowledge.[35] Second, the identification of rampant health misinformation and disinformation related to the pandemic has led platforms to take proactive measures to redirect the public. In addition to removing tweets or banning accounts promoting harmful information related to COVID-19, Twitter began labeling potentially harmful content in mid-2020 with links to curated pages with information from agencies such as the Centers for Disease Control or the World Health Organization. In January 2021, Twitter introduced Birdwatch, an approach that solicits community input to provide greater context to tweets.

Because little is known about how to measure social media impact on clinical outcomes and patient care in general, how to best leverage social media for health care delivery remains vague. As a greater percentage of the population becomes more familiar with social media and mobile devices are more accessible, there may be greater opportunities for integrating social media into patient care.

As existing social platforms adopt more features, the user interface becomes increasingly complex to navigate, raising the barrier to entry. Furthermore, as more social media platforms are developed, many health professionals may find it overwhelming to learn how to effectively use new platforms and keep up with the trends. Despite the divergence of platforms, there appears to be a convergence of features being co-opted by multiple platforms, most recently Instagram's introduction of "Reels" in response to the success of TikTok and Twitter's introduction of "Fleets" (the "stories" equivalent as seen on Instagram, Snapchat, LinkedIn, and YouTube).

To assist in the health care social media effort, many medical journals have appointed social media editors.[36] The individuals help to ensure the success of a journal's social media effort through maintaining consistency in content production, reviewing said content through a clinical lens, and engaging online audiences. Other structured efforts such as the Association for Healthcare Social Media, a 501(c)(3) nonprofit professional society for health professionals on social media, serve to provide resources in the form of tutorials and courses often in collaboration with the social media platforms themselves. Furthermore, the organization aims to raise awareness and advocate for social media use in medicine, as the benefits of social media use may not always be apparent to clinicians or their employers. There have been other parallel efforts to provide more concrete incentives to encourage social media use, such as a white paper on how to incorporate social media activity into one's curriculum vitae. The concept of social media scholarship and rubrics to measure such productivity have also been developed to potentially reward social media activity in the promotion and tenure evaluation process.[37,38]

SUMMARY

Learning to navigate a professional social media presence is not only nuanced but also constantly evolving with new social media applications and platform features. The process often begins with physicians choosing which platforms best suit their purpose and communication strengths. A comprehensive understanding of benefits of being on social media and the common pitfalls is essential to one's approach; however, more guidance and a paradigm shift to incentivized social media activity may be necessary to attract more health professionals to devote time to communicating via social media.

CLINICS CARE POINTS

- Consider delivering message via social media platforms that permit large content transmission (such as YouTube) when the goal is patient and colleague education.
- Social media platforms that rely on short communications and/or images (such as Twitter and Instagram) are better suited for announcements and relevant societal awareness.
- Refrain from debates or "back and forth" communication that can further damage professional image of posting professionals.
- If working for a large health care institution, getting to know and leveraging the existing social media editors/liaisons can help creating desired contents with professional quality.

DISCLOSURE

The author has nothing to disclose.

REFERENCES

1. Curioso WH, Proaño A, Ruiz EF. [Gastroenterology 2.0: useful resources for the gastroenterologist available on the Web 2.0]. Rev Gastroenterol Peru 2011; 31(3):245–57.
2. Kemp S. 15.5 Users Join Social Every Second (and Other Key Stats to Know). Hootsuite. 2021. Available at: https://blog.hootsuite.com/simon-kemp-social-media/. Accessed February 15, 2021.
3. Reich J, Guo L, Groshek J, et al. Social media use and preferences in patients with inflammatory bowel disease. Inflamm Bowel Dis 2019;25(3):587–91.
4. Chowdhary TS, Thompson J, Gayam S. Social media use for inflammatory bowel disease in a rural appalachian population. Telemed J E Health 2020. https://doi.org/10.1089/tmj.2020.0014.
5. Reich J, Guo L, Hall J, et al. A survey of social media use and preferences in patients with inflammatory bowel disease. Inflamm Bowel Dis 2016;22(11):2678–87.
6. Bilal M, Simons M, Rahman AU, et al. What constitutes urgent endoscopy? A social media snapshot of gastroenterologists' views during the COVID-19 pandemic. Endosc Int Open 2020;8(5):E693–8.
7. Ajumobi AB, Malakouti M, Bullen A, et al. YouTube™ as a source of instructional videos on bowel preparation: a content analysis. J Cancer Educ 2016;31(4): 755–9.
8. Aydin MF, Aydin MA. Quality and reliability of information available on YouTube and Google pertaining gastroesophageal reflux disease. Int J Med Inform 2020;137:104107.
9. Twitter. Quarterly Report. Available at: https://investor.twitterinc.com/financial-information/quarterly-results/default.aspx. Accessed February 15, 2021.

10. Chiang AL, Vartabedian B, Spiegel B. Harnessing the hashtag: a standard approach to GI dialogue on social media. Am J Gastroenterol 2016;111(8): 1082–4.
11. Facebook. Insights to go. Available at: https://www.facebook.com/iq/insights-to-go/2740m-facebook-monthly-active-users-were-2740m-as-of-september-30. Accessed February 16, 2021.
12. Brittain K, Pennings Kamp KJ, Salaysay Z. Colorectal cancer awareness for women via Facebook: a pilot study. Gastroenterol Nurs 2018;41(1):14–8.
13. Instagram. About us. Available at: https://about.instagram.com/about-us. Accessed February 15, 2021.
14. Andrew S. Nurses and doctors are flocking to TikTok to crack jokes and lip sync. But are they eroding patients' trust?. 2020. Available at: https://www.cnn.com/2020/01/18/us/tiktok-doctors-nurses-trnd/index.html. Accessed February 15, 2021.
15. Rannard G. Unprofessional TikTok medical videos 'not the norm'. *BBC News* blog. 2020. Available at: https://www.bbc.com/news/blogs-trending-51149991.
16. Basch CH, Hillyer GC, Jaime C. COVID-19 on TikTok: harnessing an emerging social media platform to convey important public health messages. Int J Adolesc Med Health 2020. https://doi.org/10.1515/ijamh-2020-0111.
17. Smith ZL, Chiang AL, Bowman D, et al. Longitudinal relationship between social media activity and article citations in the journal Gastrointestinal Endoscopy. Gastrointest Endosc 2019;90(1):77–83.
18. Fox SaD, Maeve. Health Online 2013. 2013. Available at: https://www.pewresearch.org/internet/2013/01/15/health-online-2013/. Accessed February 15, 2021.
19. Blendon RJ, Benson JM, Hero JO. Public trust in physicians–U.S. medicine in international perspective. N Engl J Med 2014;371(17):1570–2.
20. Luo M, Hao Y, Tang M, et al. Application of a social media platform as a patient reminder in the treatment of Helicobacter pylori. Helicobacter 2020;25(2):e12682.
21. Lee TH, Kim SE, Park KS, et al. Medical professionals' review of YouTube videos pertaining to exercises for the constipation relief. Korean J Gastroenterol 2018; 72(6):295–303.
22. Radadiya D, Gonzalez-Estrada A, Lira-Vera JE, et al. Colonoscopy videos on YouTube: are they a good source of patient education? Endosc Int Open 2020; 8(5):E598–606.
23. Segal JP, Abbasi F, Kanagasundaram C, et al. Does the Internet promote the unregulated use of fecal microbiota transplantation: a potential public health issue? Clin Exp Gastroenterol 2018;11:179–83.
24. Haber N, Smith ER, Moscoe E, et al. Causal language and strength of inference in academic and media articles shared in social media (CLAIMS): A systematic review. PLoS One 2018;13(5):e0196346.
25. Chiang AL, Galler Rabinowitz L, Kumar A, et al. Association between institutional social media involvement and gastroenterology divisional rankings: cohort study. J Med Internet Res 2019;21(9):e13345.
26. Natter M. Web Exclusive. Annals graphic medicine - Progress notes: How is residency? Ann Intern Med 2019;171(6):W29–30.
27. Natter M. Web Exclusive. Annals graphic medicine - Progress notes: 24-hour call. Ann Intern Med 2019;171(4):W11–2.
28. Roland D, Spurr J, Cabrera D. Preliminary Evidence for the Emergence of a Health Care Online Community of Practice: Using a Netnographic Framework for Twitter Hashtag Analytics. J Med Internet Res 2017;19(7):e252.

29. Rashid MA, Yip SWL, Gill D, et al. Sharing is caring: an analysis of #FOAMed Twitter posts during the COVID-19 pandemic. Postgrad Med J 2020. https://doi.org/10.1136/postgradmedj-2020-139267.

30. Chiang AL, Agarwal AK, Yang AY, et al. Sa1055 shifts in perspectives of social media in GI training: a three-year follow-up of a national survey of fellowship program directors. Gastroenterology 2020;158(6). S-260.

31. Shimkhada R, Attai D, Scheitler AJ, et al. Using a Twitter chat to rapidly identify barriers and policy solutions for metastatic breast cancer care: qualitative study. JMIR Public Health Surveill 2021;7(1):e23178.

32. Ojo A, Guntuku SC, Zheng M, et al. How health care workers wield influence through Twitter hashtags: retrospective cross-sectional study of the gun violence and COVID-19 public health crises. JMIR Public Health Surveill 2021;7(1): e24562.

33. Ahmed W, Jagsi R, Gutheil TG, et al. Public disclosure on social media of identifiable patient information by health professionals: content analysis of Twitter data. J Med Internet Res 2020;22(9):e19746.

34. Ugarte DA, Cumberland WG, Flores L, et al. Public attitudes about COVID-19 in response to president Trump's social media posts. JAMA Netw Open 2021;4(2): e210101.

35. Bell K. Twitter is rushing to verify health experts. *Engadget blog*. 2020. Available at: https://www.engadget.com/twitter-verified-more-than-1000-health-experts-new-verification-push-170028498.html.

36. Siau K, Lui R, Mahmood S. The role of a social media editor: What to expect and tips for success. United Eur Gastroenterol J 2020;8(10):1253–7.

37. Cabrera D, Vartabedian BS, Spinner RJ, et al. More than likes and tweets: creating social media portfolios for academic promotion and tenure. J Grad Med Educ 2017;9(4):421–5.

38. Acquaviva KD, Mugele J, Abadilla N, et al. Documenting social media engagement as scholarship: a new model for assessing academic accomplishment for the health professions. J Med Internet Res 2020;22(12):e25070.

The Future of the Private Gastroenterology Practice

Aaron J. Shiels, MD, Joseph J. Vicari, MD, MBA*

KEYWORDS

- Telehealth • Ancillaries • Efficiency • Cost • Reimbursement • Hospital service
- Competing technology • Artificial intelligence

KEY POINTS

- Improving patient access and increased use of advance practice providers (APPs) are important factors for future success.
- Maximized efficiency, reduced costs, and high quality will continue to drive patients to ambulatory endoscopy centers (AECs).
- Building a successful physician–APP hospital team will improve efficiency, improve quality, and decrease physician burnout.
- Adding and expanding ancillary services will lead to increased revenue.

The most reliable way to predict the future is to create it.

—*Abraham Lincoln*

In the late 1970s, GI services began the "great migration" from the inpatient facility to the hospital outpatient department (HOPD). The final phase of this migration, from HOPD to the private practice setting, led to the creation of the modern-day GI private practice. Today's private GI practice is a multidisciplinary practice including exam rooms, ambulatory endoscopy centers (AECs), pathology, infusion services, anesthesia services, imaging centers, and pharmacy services. The creative and intellectual capital of practice leaders will help define the private GI practice of the future.

PRIVATE PRACTICE MODELS

Consolidation of private practices has occurred over the last 20 years. Consolidation will continue through large single-specialty practices and private equity ownership of practices.

Large single-specialty practices have grown through practice mergers, acquisitions, and successful recruitment.[1] Large single-specialty practices can be modeled

Conflict of Interest Statement: The authors have no conflict of interest to disclose.
Rockford Gastroenterology Associates, Ltd, 401 Roxbury Road, Rockford, IL 61107-5075, USA
* Correspondence to.
E-mail address: drvicari@rockfordgi.com

Gastrointest Endoscopy Clin N Am 31 (2021) 709–718
https://doi.org/10.1016/j.giec.2021.05.007
1052-5157/21/© 2021 Elsevier Inc. All rights reserved.
giendo.theclinics.com

as a single corporation with ancillary services or as individual business units grouped under a single corporate structure.[2]

Private equity (PE) ownership of GI practices is rapidly growing. PE is an alternative investment process consisting of capital not listed on a public exchange. It consists of funds and investors investing in private companies or buying out private companies. PE practices improve economies of scale through consolidation of services across multiple practice sites in the same city, state, and across state lines.[1] The multiple-site and multiple-state PE-backed system is an alternative to health system acquisition and may help physicians maintain control of their practices.[1]

CLINIC SERVICES
Patient Access

An essential aspect in delivering subspecialty care is patient access to the provider, including physicians and advance practice providers (APPs) (**Box 1**). Demand for GI services continues to grow, while the number of graduating fellows remains static and the retirement process of aging gastroenterologists continues.

Several strategies can be initiated to improve patient access. Open-access scheduling is an effective method to improve access. Open access requires open appointment slots in provider schedules to allow for same-day visits. Developing a symptom- and disease-based screening protocol for triage nurses allows for appropriate use of same-day slots. More creative and technologically advanced practices could develop a web-based protocol to allow direct patient scheduling. Implementing and maintaining a successful open-access model requires buy-in from triage nurses, physicians, and administration.

Provider Clinic Work

The addition of APPs to GI practices has increased over the last decade. APPs have become an important part of the inpatient and outpatient GI team. Gastroenterologists split their time between the clinic, AEC, and hospital. This splitting of time decreases availability to evaluate outpatients in the clinic setting, potentially decreasing access. The use of APPs will continue to grow. The future supply of APPs will greatly exceed the future supply of gastroenterologists. In the future, gastroenterologists will spend the majority of their time performing endoscopic procedures. Their limited time spent performing cognitive services will be focused on complex inflammatory bowel disease, hepatology, and pancreaticobiliary disease. Increasing use of APPs will improve patient access, improve quality of care, and improve clinic efficiency (**Box 2**).

The scope of practice for APPs will continue to evolve. In the future, APPs may perform flexible sigmoidoscopy, hemorrhoidal banding, trigger point injections for abdominal wall pain, and with the use of AI perhaps upper endoscopy and screening colonoscopy (see section on AI). The outcome of expanding the scope of services of

---

Box 1
Clinic services

Patient access

Provider clinic work

Subspecialty clinics

Telehealth

Box 2
Possible future scope of APP practice
Flexible sigmoidoscopy
Hemorrhoid banding
Trigger point injection
Upper endoscopy and colonoscopy using artificial intelligence

APPs will be increased professional satisfaction for APPs (diverse skill set) and increased access for certain GI services.

Subspecialty Clinic

Traditionally, GI subspecialty clinics only existed in academic centers (**Box 3**). The formation of large single-specialty practices and PE ownership of GI practices provide the resources to develop subspecialty clinics. Larger groups have the resources and patient population to recruit GI subspecialists who could focus on their cognitive and endoscopic interests. APPs could be included when developing cognitive subspecialty clinics. Private practice subspecialty clinics have the potential to improve practice efficiency, improve patient outcomes, increase patient volume, and improve professional satisfaction.

Telehealth

The COVID-19 pandemic unexpectedly caused practices to implement telehealth services. The previous impediment for telehealth implementation, inadequate reimbursement, was rapidly removed at the onset of the COVID-19 pandemic. Almost all private payors, Medicare, and Medicaid increased reimbursement for outpatient telehealth clinic evaluations on a level consistent with in-person evaluations. If reimbursement remains acceptable, telehealth will improve patient access, by providing access to GI care for patients in remote access areas and those unable to leave their home or care facility.

Telehealth has the potential to increase patient volume by promoting services to patients over a wide geographic area. Increasing access to patients over a wide geographic area has the potential to increase volume in the clinic and AEC.

AEC
Cost to Payors

The components of costs to payors and reimbursement to providers for an endoscopic procedure are the professional fee and facility fee. The professional fee is

Box 3
GI subspecialty clinics
Complex inflammatory bowel disease
Hepatology
Nonpancreaticobiliary advanced endoscopy
Functional disorders
Pancreatic biliary diseases including advanced endoscopic procedures

the same for an endoscopic procedure performed in the AEC and HOPD. However, there is a great difference in reimbursement when comparing the facility fee in the AEC and HOPD. The HOPD remains burdened by a higher facility fee compared with the AEC. AECs offer endoscopic services at a significantly lower cost compared with the HOPD for similar endoscopic services in a similarly regulated environment. The disparity in costs between the AEC and HOPD will continue to drive endoscopic procedures from the HOPD to AEC. Based on current AEC and HOPD payments, cost savings continue for payors and beneficiaries. AECs offer valuable endoscopic services at a significantly lower cost for similar services compared to HOPD.

Efficiency in the AEC

Efficiency can be planned and assessed on multiple levels and in the context of many variables when delivering endoscopic services.[3] The physical environment of an AEC should be designed to allow for efficient and safe movement of staff, patients, and family throughout the facility. A well-designed AEC maximizes efficiency, minimizes travel distance, and achieves economy of movement. In successful endoscopy units, preparation, recovery, endoscope reprocessing, and patient flow all occur efficiently and safely.

Optimize Efficiency

In assessing efficiency within endoscopy centers there are several potential areas where process improvements can be implemented: personnel utilization, patient scheduling, and procedure delays.[4]

Perhaps the most important factor affecting personnel utilization is staff number. There should be at least 1 staff member, typically an RN in each endoscopy room. Additionally, there should be a minimum of 1.5 full-time equivalent (FTEs) in prep/recovery for each active endoscopy room. A dedicated endoscope technician leads to more efficient room turnover. These technicians also assist with simple tasks during endoscopic procedures. When using dedicated endoscope technicians, one should plan on 0.5 to 0.75 FTEs per active endoscopy room. These recommendations represent minimum staffing levels. Each AEC should identify and develop staffing ratios that best meet its needs.

Block scheduling is the most efficient way to schedule endoscopic procedures. Using standard time slots (30 minutes) for endoscopic procedures allows schedulers to offer patients more options when scheduling procedures. Block scheduling also offers flexibility regarding individual physician needs during endoscopy. Implementation of a dedicated screening colonoscopy scheduler improves scheduling efficiency. It also permits improved tracking of patients within the system, leading to more effective patient counseling.

Open-access endoscopy has become common in the USA, primarily to accommodate the volume of screening procedures required by the healthy population.[3] Open-access endoscopy should have strict criteria defining patient eligibility. Once criteria have been developed and implemented, it is important to share the guidelines with referring physicians so they better understand which patients are eligible for open-access endoscopy. Also, the criteria are used by nursing staff to help screen appropriate patients for open-access endoscopy and avoid inappropriate patient scheduling. The goal of open-access endoscopy is to increase patient convenience while maintaining quality care.

It is important to minimize delays in the AEC. There are two types of delays in the AEC, patient and procedure related.[4] Management strategies can be employed to decrease patient delays in the AEC. These include ensuring patient instructions are clear, providing accurate directions to the AEC, performing an advance call to patients to review preparatory instructions/medications, and ensuring an efficient check-in process once the patient arrives at the AEC.[4] Procedure-related delays are most often related to physicians. Physician-related delays are typically the result of multitasking, performing tasks unrelated to endoscopy, and intraprocedure physician delays.[4] Physician-related delays in the AEC should be monitored and redirected by physician leaders.[4]

ANCILLARY SERVICES

Reduced reimbursement for GI procedures increases economic pressure on private GI practices. Simultaneously, increased practice expenses and regulatory burdens create additional stress. Adding ancillary services can increase revenue and improve the financial health of the organization. Ancillary services also offer opportunities for improved quality and efficiency within the practice. The following sections review the potential upside and downside of ancillary services.

Anesthesia Services

Utilization of anesthesia services has steadily increased over the last two decades. Currently, more than half of all endoscopic procedures utilize monitored anesthesia care (MAC),[5] typically administered by an anesthesiologist or certified registered nurse anesthetist. Many practices have incorporated anesthesia services into their AEC model, thus providing another source of revenue. There are 3 options by which anesthesia services can be incorporated in the private practice AEC setting. In all cases, consultation with a healthcare attorney is essential to avoid violation of evolving laws and regulations.

The first option is to establish 100% ownership in the anesthesia group, often established as a separate limited liability corporation (LLC). This option allows the practice to retain control of daily operations, employment of anesthesia providers, billing, and collections. Anesthesia providers can be employees of the LLC or contracted on a 1099 basis. This option allows the practice the greatest control over cost and quality of anesthesia services. This arrangement may carry the highest risk of violation of Stark laws or regulations that aim to limit self-referral.

The second option is to enter into a joint venture with an anesthesia management corporation. The practice can obtain an additional revenue stream, while ceding control of daily operations and anesthesia provider employment to the anesthesia management company. Many of the burdensome compliance issues would be unloaded also.

The third option is to contract with an outside anesthesia provider. Most of the compliance and employment issues are managed by the anesthesia group, who also handle billing and collections. The major disadvantage is much of the additional revenue is captured by the outside anesthesia group, unless a revenue-sharing process is established. This approach may be used by practices that perform most of the procedures with moderate sedation but need propofol for a small subset of patients.

Although there is a need for MAC in certain patient groups, debate continues as to whether the use of MAC anesthesia is appropriate for all low-risk patients.[6] This could potentially be an issue in the future despite the growing utilization of anesthesia services for GI procedures.[7] Although use of MAC may improve AEC efficiency through faster sedation and recovery periods, there is no strong evidence that patient outcomes or safety are improved when compared to moderate sedation. There is significant geographic variation in the use of anesthesia services, however it cannot be considered standard of care. It is possible there will be additional downward pressures on reimbursement for anesthesia services. Practices using moderate sedation may maintain a competitive advantage by providing a lower overall cost of colonoscopy. This may be attractive to integrative healthcare networks searching for lower cost endoscopy services. Local and regional market forces may determine whether anesthesia services are financially acceptable.

Pathology

AECs generate pathology specimens that require processing and analysis. This provides an opportunity to improve quality, shorten turnaround, and create an additional revenue stream by insourcing pathology services. This can be accomplished by insourcing the technical component (TC), professional component (PC), or both. Practices considering in-house pathology services should generate an adequate number of specimens to allow recoupment of initial capital outlay and ongoing costs. Smaller practices (less than 5000 specimens yearly) are probably best served by sending their specimens to an outside pathology lab.

Specimens are fixed in formalin and processed for reading by the pathologist. This is the TC of the pathology service. Practices opting to insource the TC are reimbursed by Medicare and commercial insurance for this service. The initial capital costs include building the lab, purchasing equipment, and hiring a consultant to assist with planning and legal/regulatory issues. There are operational expenses including supplies, maintenance/repair of equipment, and salary for a histopathology technician. In a busy practice, the startup costs can generally be recouped within a year and the TC alone can be an excellent ancillary revenue source.

Analysis and generation of a report by a pathologist comprise the PC, generating a second fee. For practices that solely insource the TC, the pathology slides are sent to an outside pathologist for interpretation. The PC fee is not captured by the practice. If this service is provided by an in-house pathologist, the practice captures the PC also. Many practices have opted to insource the PC with an employed pathologist or one working as an independent contractor.

There are several important factors for practices considering adding pathology services. The most important is to ensure adequate procedure volume exists, generating enough specimens to make it financially viable. Practices should also work closely with a consultant and healthcare attorney who can navigate the complex rules and regulations at both the federal and state levels. Although in-office ancillary exceptions to the Stark law generally allow in-house pathology services, it is important to fully understand these issues before committing to the project. For practices utilizing in-house pathologists, hiring a pathologist with specific GI training can significantly enhance the quality of patient care.

Infusion Center

Inflammatory bowel disease is increasingly treated with medications that require regular infusions. Traditionally, patients have been infused at hospital outpatient infusion centers. Recently, payors have changed coverage to require infusions be performed elsewhere due to the high costs associated with hospital outpatient infusion centers. Options for infusion sites include home infusion, free-standing infusion centers, and office-based infusion centers. Increasingly, private GI practices are adding office-based infusion centers as an ancillary service.[8]

GI practice-owned and -operated infusion centers offer several advantages. Coordination of care is optimized as patients receive infusions with direct oversight by the managing gastroenterologist. Scheduling is controlled by the practice. This arrangement improves compliance and patient satisfaction. Payors previously reimbursing at higher charges associated with hospital outpatient infusion centers recognize the value provided by the lower cost office-based infusion centers. It also provides an important ancillary revenue stream for the GI practice. In order for an infusion center to become financially successful, there should be an adequate volume of patients receiving regular infusions.

The startup costs associated with an infusion center include construction costs, supplies, information technology, and setup. Because of the high acquisition cost of medications, it is essential to have a thorough understanding of all financial factors. Medications are typically obtained through direct purchasing arrangements with wholesalers prior to infusion. Reimbursement from payors may occur up to 90 days after infusion. Therefore, there may be a significant capital outlay at the onset. Payment covers medication costs and infusion services. Management can be performed by the practice or by contracting with an outside infusion management company. A busy infusion center can provide an excellent source of revenue while improving patient satisfaction.

Imaging

Improved patient satisfaction and better care coordination may lead a GI practice to consider adding imaging services. The decision to incorporate an imaging center depends on volume of imaging studies and reimbursement. CT, MRI, ultrasound, and vibration-controlled elastography (VCTE) are imaging modalities that could be offered.

There is substantial capital investment for initial construction and equipment. In the case of CT and MRI, the costs can exceed $1 to 2 million. Ultrasound and VCTE equipment can be obtained for more modest investments. It is important to determine volume, charges, payor mix, and any ongoing costs prior to finalizing a plan.

With the exception of VCTE, which can be interpreted by a gastroenterologist, the other imaging modalities require a radiologist for interpretation. There are several models available, each with its own advantages. One model allows the radiologist to read and collect professional fees. The practice can negotiate a contract allowing a percentage of the fees to be retained by the practice. Another option, if there is sufficient volume, is to employ a radiologist. As with other ancillary services, it is important to consult a healthcare attorney to avoid any legal or regulatory issues at the federal and state levels.

Pharmacy

Improved compliance, higher patient satisfaction, and an additional revenue stream are reasons to consider the addition of in-office pharmacy. The convenience associated with picking up prescriptions at the same visit can lead to improved compliance and patient satisfaction. There is typically no associated physician time involved and the increased revenue can be significant. The costs associated with an in-office pharmacy include developing physical space with any required equipment and employing a licensed pharmacist or pharmacy technician. It is important to assess prescription volumes to maintain adequate inventory. Most states have regulations that permit in-office medication dispensing only for patients cared for by the practice.

HOSPITAL SERVICE—THE APP/PHYSICIAN TEAM

The use of APPs, including nurse practitioners and physician assistants, has steadily increased in private GI practices.[9] The advantages of employing APPs include improved access to patient care, freeing up physicians to concentrate on complex patients and procedures, decreased physician burnout, and enhanced revenue to the practice. APPs are utilized in outpatient clinics, inpatient hospital services, or a combination of these two settings.[6]

The diagnoses and patient acuity encountered in the inpatient setting require a special skill set. Inpatient APPs will typically consult on patients in collaboration with an attending physician. Other responsibilities include daily rounding on inpatients, scheduling of procedures, ordering tests, arranging discharge, and coordinating outpatient follow=up. In many ways, the hospital-based APP manages the inpatient service, allowing the physician to focus on procedures and more complex patient care issues. It is essential to establish a strong, collegial working relationship between the APP and physician.

A successful relationship starts with establishing appropriate expectations for the APP. For APPs with GI experience, a busy service with high inpatient load may be easily managed. However, many APPs will come directly from training with no experience managing complex GI conditions. In this case, an orientation/training period is essential. This allows the physician or more experienced APP to assist in the education of the new APP. The APP steadily gains experience and confidence in diagnosis and management. The orientation period also fosters a strong working relationship and compatibility between the APP and physician. This team becomes an efficient machine, providing high-quality inpatient GI services. Patient and referring physician satisfaction are typically excellent because of accessibility, continuity of care, and overall high-quality service provided by a team approach.

BUNDLED SERVICES

Controlling rising healthcare costs in the USA remains a high priority. Although the traditional fee-for-service model is still the predominant payment method, other options to provide high-quality, value-based care have emerged. Bundled payment for well-defined episodes of care is a promising option. However, widespread adoption has not been realized.

Both screening and diagnostic colonoscopy can be effectively incorporated into a bundled payment contract.[10–12] Colonoscopy is a well-defined episode with preoperative, intraoperative, and postoperative phases. The associated costs are easy to identify and control. Private practices with an AEC have a significant advantage over hospitals when negotiating bundled contracts because of the low-cost, high-quality setting. The GI practice can leverage this advantage to develop contracts with various payors. The payment arrangement covers all costs associated with colonoscopy, including professional and facility fees. The bundle price typically includes any preprocedure assessment, bowel prep, colonoscopy procedure including sedation/anesthesia, pathology TC and PC fees, and any necessary follow-up within the postprocedure interval. Whether complications are included is subject to negotiation. This arrangement can be particularly attractive to self-insured employers seeking well-defined costs and high-quality services.

There are important considerations when developing and negotiating a bundled payment contract. It is important to determine the historical utilization for the particular patient population that would be covered by the bundled contract. This information is essential to negotiating a fair final bundled price for colonoscopy. The bundled contract needs to address situations that occur infrequently such as incomplete procedures, multiple procedures, complications, and procedures that need to be repeated (such as large polyps). Finally, because utilization of anesthesia services varies from practice to practice, the percentage of procedures with anesthesia will impact the final bundled price. Practices that utilize moderate sedation for average-risk patients have a competitive cost advantage when negotiating a bundled payment contract.

COMPETITIVE TECHNOLOGIES

Colonoscopy is the most commonly performed procedure at AECs. Of these colonoscopies, the majority are performed for the purposes of colon cancer screening and polyp surveillance. As a result of this procedure volume, colonoscopy is the primary source of revenue for AECs. If a significant decrease in colonoscopy volume occurs, this could threaten the financial viability of AECs. Potential competitive technologies could emerge in the coming years. The most likely threat to colonoscopy as a screening test for colon cancer is the multitarget stool DNA with fecal immunochemical testing (MT-sDNA).

MT-sDNA is a noninvasive test used to screen for colon cancer. The noninvasive nature of MT-sDNA makes it appealing to patients and easier to perform compared with colonoscopy. Potentially, it may be easier for primary care physicians to promote use of MT-sDNA to patients compared with colonoscopy. Although colonoscopy is the recommended screening test for colon cancer compared to MT-sDNA, increased use of the MT-sDNA test has the potential to decrease colonoscopy volume in AECs and therefore decrease AEC revenue. Private practice groups should monitor incoming screening colonoscopy referrals, assessing for a decrease in referrals. The monitoring process should also assess the number of colonoscopies performed for a positive MT-sDNA test. Practices should access education material from the GI societies to develop a local colon cancer screening education process to promote the value of colonoscopy compared with other screening tests.

ARTIFICIAL INTELLIGENCE

Artificial intelligence (AI) holds tremendous promise to augment clinical performance, establish better treatment plans, and improve patient outcomes.[13] Although the initial experience is encouraging for AI in gastroenterology, there are currently many uncertainties. AI refers to the ability of a computer to perform a task associated with intelligent beings, including cognitive function that might mimic the human mind, such as the ability to learn.[14] In GI, AI has potential practical applications in both cognitive and endoscopic aspects of clinical practice. The role of AI in the private practice GI group will emerge in the coming years. Important questions for practice leadership to consider regarding the use of AI within private practice include: logistics of implementation and use, cost of implementing AI, who will use AI, what roles AI will have in cognitive practice, and what role AI will have in endoscopic practice. Despite the unknown future of AI, the initial data within GI are promising and exciting.

SUMMARY

The future private gastroenterology practice will be a large multidisciplinary practice including a clinic, AEC, pathology services, infusion services, anesthesia services, pharmacy services, and imaging centers. Delivery of GI services will be a team-based clinic with AEC access and improvement of quality of care. Competing technologies will drive practices to promote the value of colonoscopy as the best screening test for colon cancer. AI may significantly alter our approach to clinic and endoscopic services. The creative and intellectual capital of practice leaders will continue to define the private GI practice of the future.

CLINICS CARE POINTS

- APP's are an essential part of the GI clinical team.
- ASC's provide efficient and quality endoscopic services.
- Office based infusion services provide cost effective care for patients and payors.
- Bundled contracts can increase patient volume and generate new source of revenue.

REFERENCES

1. Allen JI, Kaushal N. New models of gastroenterology practice. Clin Gastroenterol Hepatol 2018;16:3–6.
2. Pallardy C. 7 gastroenterologists leading GI mega practices. Beckers GII and Endoscopy. 2015. https://www.beckersAEC.com/gastroenterology-and-endoscopy/5-gastroenterologists-leading-gi-mega-practices.html. Accessed January 2021. Google.
3. Peterson BT. Promoting efficiency in gastrointestinal endoscopy. Gastrointest Endosc Clin N Am 2006;16(4):671–85.
4. Day LW, Belson D. Studying and incorporating efficiency into gastrointestinal endoscopy centers. Gastroenterol Res Pract 2015;2015:764153.
5. Khiani VS, Soulos P, Gancayco J. Anesthesiologist involvement in screening colonoscopy: temporal trends and cost implications for the Medicare population. Clin Gastroenterol Hepatol 2012;10:58–64.
6. Early DS, Lightdale JH, Vargo JJ. Guidelines for sedation and anesthesia in GI endoscopy. Gastrointest Endosc 2018;87:327–37.
7. Inadomi JM, Gunnarsson CL, Rizzo JA. Projected increased growth rate of anesthesia professional-delivered sedation for colonoscopy and EGD in the United States from 2009-2015. Gastrointest Endosc 2010;72:580–6.
8. Managing an in-office infusion practice, The Rheumatologist. Available at: http://www.the-rheumatologist.org/article/managing-an-in-office-infusion-practice. Accessed March 12, 2020.
9. Nandwani MC, Clark JO. Incorporating advanced practice providers into gastroenterology practice. Clin Gastroenterol Hepatol 2019;17:365–9.
10. Allen JI, Aldrich L, Moote M. Building a team-based gastroenterology practice with advanced practice providers. Gastroenterol Hepatol 2019;15:213–20.
11. Ketover SR. Bundled payment for colonoscopy. Frontline Medical Communications: GI and Hepatology News; 2013.
12. Brill JV, Jain R, Margolis PS. A bundled payment framework for colonoscopy performed for colorectal cancer screening or surveillance. Gastroenterology 2014; 146:849–53.
13. Berzin TM, Parasa S, Wallace MB, et al. Position statement on priorities for artificial intelligence in GI endoscopy: a report by the ASGE Task Force. Gastrointest Endosc 2020;92(4):951–9.
14. Russell SJ, Norvig P. Artificial intelligence, a modern approach. Upper Saddle River, New Jersey: Pearson Education; 2009.

Developing Endoscopic Services in a Large Health Care System

John J. Vargo, MD, MPH, MASGE, FGJES[a,b,c,d,e,*]

KEYWORDS

- Endoscopy operation • Health care reimbursement model,
- Multidisciplinary patient care

KEY POINTS

- Rising costs in the United States mandated the need for value-based reimbursement approach for health care services.
- Endoscopy operations must reflect the value-based model by providing a wide array of endoscopic services in a cost-effective manner.
- All facets of revenue generation and cost containment for endoscopic services are best obtained when an organization specific, multidisciplinary approach – inclusive of different medical disciplines, institutional administration and ancillary staffs - is implemented.
- The proper governance of an enterprise endoscopic service in a large health care system requires a clearly defined reporting structure and collaboration among clinical and nonclinical members for transparent accountability.

INTRODUCTION

Health care spending is projected to grow at an average rate of nearly 6% per year from 2018 to 2027.[1] In addition, it is expected to reach nearly $6 trillion in expenditures by 2027. This represents an increase in the fraction of health care's effect on the gross domestic product from 17.9% in 2017 to 19.4% by 2027. The merger and affiliation activity of hospitals, physician groups, and other health care organizations adds another layer of complexity to the health care space. The shift from fee-for-service to value-based care continues, and with this comes the goal to provide high quality and valuable patient care while at the same time keeping pace with innovation to continuously improve the practice of medicine.

The health service line concept for gastrointestinal disorders (GI) requires a coordinated approach focusing on high clinical quality, outstanding patient satisfaction, and

[a] Enterprise Endoscopy Operations; [b] Endoscopic Research and Innovation; [c] Section of Advanced Endoscopy; [d] Department of Gastroenterology, Hepatology and Nutrition; [e] Digestive Disease and Surgery Institute, Cleveland Clinic, Cleveland, OH, USA
* 9500 Euclid Avenue A-31, Cleveland, OH 44195.
E-mail address: vargoj@ccf.org

Gastrointest Endoscopy Clin N Am 31 (2021) 719–725
https://doi.org/10.1016/j.giec.2021.05.008
1052-5157/21/© 2021 Elsevier Inc. All rights reserved.

giendo.theclinics.com

developing and delivering innovation, all at an appropriate cost structure to attract payers and thereby boost patient volumes further. Although many health care systems have focused on reducing expenses, realignment of health care delivery could lead to a cost reduction of up to 25%.[2]

The development of the concept of endoscopy operations for the author's institution became an imperative step to evolve out of the traditional department-based model of care as endoscopic practice involved both gastroenterologists and surgical endoscopists. Sites of service within the organization were varied. These included hospital-based endoscopic centers, ambulatory surgery centers, and ambulatory endoscopy centers. Each of these site types developed their own operational cadence and microcultures. The standardization of procedural policies, equipment, competency, and personnel management remains an imperative step to deliver value-based care. In addition, the development of overall mission statement, governance structure, and strategy were necessary to further coordinate efforts. This article discusses the endoscopy operation model adopted in the author's institution to provide comprehensive and efficient care of a wide array of endoscopic service.

HOW TO STRUCTURE A SERVICE LINE

In order to optimize the disease centered product line, the author found that the traditional department model did not suffice in many circumstances, owing to the fact that endoscopic services are provided by medical and surgical departments. In order to optimize value-based delivery of services, the traditional departmental approach made way for a coordinated effort along disease-centered patient care pathways. There are different blueprints to consider when building a disease-based product line.

The service line organization model finds itself organized around the service lines themselves. This works best in organizations that have abandoned the traditional departmental governance model and instead focused their efforts around a cluster of system- or organ-specific disease processes.

A service line marketing model utilizes marketing strategy to grow specific service lines. This model is limited by the fact that there is no direct linkage to medical operations.

The service line leadership model uses the service line leader for product line development and strategic goals. As with the service line marketing model, the lack of medical operations dimension limits systemwide implementation of value-based care through cost containment and quality improvement. The service line management model uses a service line manager who is directly responsible for day-to-day operations, quality improvement, and service line growth in product line cost management. The service line organizational model offers the highest ability to bring about change but also has a steeper implementation curve. Many health care organizations use a hybridization of 2 models in order to optimize governance, value-based care, and growth.[3]

Another important concept is that of developing a portfolio of differentiated service line capabilities across the across the health system with respect to endoscopic services. Whenever possible, complex, high-cost and labor-intensive procedures such as endoscopic retrograde cholangiopancreatography (ERCP), endoscopic submucosal dissection, Peroral endoscopic myotomy (POEM), G-POEM, and third space endoscopy should be focused in centers of excellence where teams are specially developed to carry out these procedures and the address acuity of the patients themselves. Utilizing a wheel and spoke model, procedures of lesser complexity are performed at ambulatory surgical centers and ambulatory endoscopy centers, often located in regional centers, in contrast to the main hub. In health systems with multiple hospitals, ultrahigh complexity cases among particularly high acuity patients may further be directed toward a single center (the main hub) in order to optimize outcomes. In addition, it makes little sense to develop a bariatric endoscopy program without having located in the same building as the bariatric surgery, nutritional, and medical obesity specialists. Colocation of like-minded medical and surgical services improves patient satisfaction by providing convenience and a multidisciplinary care.

Other key components when developing and managing an endoscopy product line include the development of a physician/administrator leadership team known as a dyad.[4] This important leadership unit within the table of organization of a GI endoscopy product line allows for a broader approach to the complexity encountered with the often complementary expertise of the leadership dyad. The governance and organizational structure of the service line is also of a critical importance. This will be more thoroughly outlined. But physicians, administrators, nurses, scheduling personnel and technicians, and other ancillary services such as human physiology need to be included in this table of organization in order to optimize stakeholder input. Perhaps one of the biggest challenges of such an endeavor is appropriate amalgamation of cultures among stakeholders, institutions, and other practice sites to create a collaborative organization that is focused on the primary mission of the enterprise endoscopy product line. It is important to gain a deep understanding of the financial and operational aspects of the service line that will result in minimizing cost per case while at the same time maximizing quality outcomes. Understanding and managing the product line's data to drive quality outcomes and minimize costs are also important factors. Additionally, identifying and training future leaders in the organizational structure from the decision, nursing, and administrative standpoint are important in succession planning.

STRATEGIC DEVELOPMENT OF ENDOSCOPIC PROCEDURES

Strategic addition of new procedures to the existing endoscopic practice is key to promulgating a cycle of innovation and providing quality care to the patient population. It is also an important avenue for attracting faculty and developing the careers of existing endoscopists. As new technologies and procedures are developed, it is important that the organization review these for their potential merit in patient care by replacing other procedures or filling a void. For example, the development of endoscopic submucosal dissection at the author's institution has led to the development of a center for the evaluation and management of superficial mucosal malignancies of the foregut and hindgut.

One can consider developing a committee that is focused on the review and adoption of new endoscopic procedures. This requires a business review with the identification of possible patients who may benefit from the procedure. Once this has been accomplished, the appropriate recruitment of new faculty or training of existing faculty is then necessary. Typically, the introduction of these procedures is done at one of the major centers of quaternary and tertiary care. The volume and outcomes are assessed frequently and when the quantity and quality of the procedures reach a certain threshold, expansion of the procedures at the established sites and consideration of scalability of the procedures throughout the endoscopic practice enterprise are considered.

ENTERPRISE ENDOSCOPY OPERATIONS GOVERNANCE

There are a multitude of governance organizational structures. A specific organizational structure can be standardized for the needs of the enterprise. The author's practice utilizes a dyad of a physician and administrator to oversee endoscopic operations.[5] The dyad reports to the institute chair – administrator dyad. The author's practice employs a standing committee structure, and when needed, ad hoc task forces for issues that either require the input of 2 or more of the standing committees or stakeholders outside of the governance stricture. Given the size and geographic diversity of the enterprise, essentially all of the meetings are held on a virtual platform (**Fig. 1**).

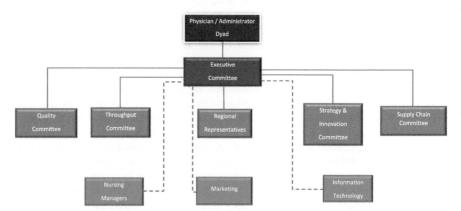

Fig. 1. Endoscopy operations table of organization. *Solid lines* represent a primary/direct line of report. *Dashed lines* represent a secondary line of report.

The keys to successful governance structure include

Inclusivity: stakeholder representation is crucial to ensure that a balanced perspective on each issue is achieved; all members of the committees are able to bring forth agenda items

Transparency: meeting minutes are distributed and when necessary, communiques in the form of E-mails and presentations at department meetings are used

Action item closure: the key to a successful committee environment is active discussion, the development of action items, and the successful completion of those action items at a later executive committee meeting

Executive Committee

Chaired by the endoscopy operations physician-administrator dyad, the executive committee members include the chairs of the throughput, supply chain, quality, strategy, and innovations committees, as well as representation from the anesthesia department and nursing. Additionally, the chairpersons of the digestive disease and surgery institute and the department of gastroenterology and hepatology are members. Regional representation is also included by geographic region. Meetings are held in a designated frequency and include the reports from the committee chairpersons, regional leaders, and nursing and anesthesia staff based on an appropriate agenda and goal.

Throughput Committee

The throughput committee is charged with optimizing patient flow through the various endoscopy units. It also ensures that policies for other elements such as personal protective equipment and staffing ratios are adhered to. The committee is composed of physicians, nurses, and front desk and scheduling personnel. This committee meets weekly in our institution.

Supply Chain Committee

The supply chain committee is composed of physicians, nurses, administrators, and supply chain representatives. The committee has several charges. One of these is contract negotiation with vendors. This is done on a cyclical basis, every 3 to 4 years. Vendor fairs are held so that there is input on potential additions to the equipment portfolio by physicians and nursing staff. Another important function of the committee is the evaluation of new accessories and equipment. Vendors are not allowed to introduce equipment into the organization without this evaluation process, which includes the identification of a physician. Typically, a physician sponsor will bring a proposal to the committee regarding a particular accessory or piece of equipment. The committee assesses the value of this accessory to the practice: does it replace an existing piece of equipment in a cost-effective fashion, or does it represent a new treatment option? If the latter is apparent, the strategy committee will render an opinion. If approved for evaluation, the committee and physician sponsor will identify a group of physicians to try the product. Once the trial is completed, the physician champion will then report to the supply chain committee with the results. The committee will then vote on adding the accessory to the inventory and consider removing existing pieces of equipment that the new device would replace. On the committee, conflict of interest is taken seriously and with transparency. The members of the committee who have relationships with the vendors under discussion must be recused from the discussion and subsequent voting.

Quality Committee

The charges of this committee include assuring that practice within the product line follows evidence-based medicine and provisions that ensure that timely and accurate documentation of clinical and procedural notes is maintained. The quality committee should also assure that the appropriate credentialing and certification of each member of the endoscopy operations team is maintained and that each endoscopy unit conforms to a universal approach to endoscope reprocessing. The quality committee is also charged with reviewing any instances where there may have been a deviation in practice in providing remediation and/or recommendations of policy changes as necessary. The quality committee also develops an endoscopy report card for each practitioner. In its most basic form, quality outcomes for upper endoscopy and colonoscopy such as cecal intubation rate, adenoma detection rate, and photo-documentation of landmarks should be included. More sophisticated analyses such as cost per case after adjustment for complexity can also be addressed. The chairperson of the quality committee is also the endoscopy product line's quality officer. In some organizations, the quality committee is also charged with conducting morbidity and mortality rounds, wherein cases are presented with the purpose of reviewing management decisions and how to optimize care for patients in the future.

Strategy and Innovation Committee

The charge of the strategy and innovation committee provides the executive committee with a landscape snapshot of developments in GI endoscopy and recommends which avenues should be explored to add to the endoscopy enterprise's diagnostic and therapeutic armamentarium. In addition, the committee provides information on the scalability of certain procedures to additional practice sites by employing a comprehensive business analysis. In the case of innovative procedures, existing faculty may be earmarked for innovation trips to learn the procedures from existing sites around the globe. Alternatively, faculty may be hired to develop this product line.

TRACKING METRICS

Developing a report card that includes finance, patient satisfaction, clinical outcomes, and efficiency measures is extremely important. Continuously addressing patient access is a central tenet of performance measurement. A key component to this is setting a time threshold for elective staff time away so that the interval between the threshold and patient access is wide enough so that scheduling occurs to fill the white space within the schedule. A periodic endoscopy operations meeting that includes physicians and nursing and support staff should address this in order to optimize any downtime. In the author's institution, 95% slot utilization rate is the goal.

Developing a triage policy to ensure that emergent and urgent cases are appropriately scheduled is also important. The author has found that an elective outpatient Saturday endoscopy schedule at the ambulatory endoscopy units is popular. In addition, opening the hospital endoscopy units on Saturday leads to injured decreased length of stay and can minimize urgent and emergent procedures off hours. Tracking a patient's journey through the individual endoscopy units can be rewarding. Tracking on time starts and room turnover has been shown to optimize patient throughput. Tracking procedural volume by site, procedure type, and provider can provide insight into the overall dynamics of the endoscopic practice. Upward trends and growth for particular centers may result in adding more providers to that site. In addition, downward trending volumes need to be analyzed for potential causes such as decreases in patient satisfaction and inability to schedule at that site or shifts in the competitive landscape. Ultimately, developing a cost per case metric should be the goal for most uncomplicated procedures. It is important, however, to ensure that the level of complexity is included in this calculation, as well as any complications or unexpected hospitalizations.

Tracking the use of each scope in the endoscopic inventory, as well as a repair history, can give an insight into which instruments may need to be replaced. The author has adopted a proactive schedule wherein planned purchases of endoscopic equipment are placed in the budget. This minimizes the unplanned purchase of equipment but does not eliminate it altogether. Additionally, the enterprise endoscopy inventory database allows the replacement of endoscopes at 1 site with underutilized endoscopes at another, thereby reducing costs. By continually monitoring performance, the endoscopic product line can benchmark itself against past performance and national norms and demonstrate its value.

Information Technology

Information technology (IT) is a mission critical aspect of any endoscopy operations service to uphold fidelity of data and a foundation of patient record privacy and access. The author's institute has an embedded IT advisor and a separate electronic medical records representative who help with selecting new products, software upgrades, and solving temporary platform outages or underperformance. Both of IT and EMR representatives serve on selected committees such as throughput and strategy on an as needed basis.

Promotion of the Service Line

External promotion of the product line is important for the expansion and continued growth of endoscopic service. One of the best ways to achieve this task is to focus communication through participation at national meetings and publications in peer-reviewed journals.[6] At national meetings, advances in care and technique can be show-cased through the presentation of abstracts and participation at postgraduate courses. In the era of the coronavirus disease 2019 pandemic, use of webinars has greatly enhanced the bandwidth for national and international participation. The use of E-mails and mailings can be used on a national, regional, and local level in order to showcase key elements of the endoscopy product line portfolio along with contact information.

If an organization has a communications liaison, one should take full advantage of this opportunity and meet periodically with this person or department. This allows an institution to develop a communications strategy on upcoming events key developments in endoscopic care and focus referring doctors and the public to new procedures or faculty additions. Of course, social media are powerful tool and have been covered previously in this issue.

CONCLUSIONS

In conclusion, the development of an enterprise endoscopy operations service line carries with it the distinct advantages of practice standardization and the potential for strategic growth. As health care organizations continue a shift toward value-based care, developing a governance structure that is flexible, inclusive, and scalable will ensure continued success.

CLINICS CARE POINTS

- Consider converting to a service line-centered approach of endoscopic service in order to adopt to the value-based care reimbursement more efficiently.

- When implementing service line model approach for enterprise endoscopic operation, consult with potential stakeholders in order to develop standardized care paths, quality metrics, and referral patterns before execution.

- Leveraging the internal IT department and social media liaison is crucial for seamless data collection and promotion of existing endoscopic service lines.

DISCLOSURE

Consultant: Docbot, Exact Sciences Advisory Board: AsperoMedical.

REFERENCES

1. Available at: https://www.cms.gov/Research-Statistics-Data-and-Systems/Statistics-Trends-and-Reports/NationalHealthExpendData/Downloads/ForecastSummary.pdf.
2. Porter ME, Teisberg EO. Redefining healthcare: creating value based competition depending on results. Boston (MA): Harvard Business Review Press; 2006.
3. Available at: https://www.beckershopstialreview.com/hosptials-key specialties/4-models-for structures-for structuring-a-service-line. Accessed March 5, 2021.
4. Biga C, Blanknship JC, Campbell R, et al. Developing and managing a successful CV service line. https://www.acc.org/~/media/14B6F431FBC24192A316DD3DFAF34780.ashx.
5. Zismer PK, Brueggemann J. Examining the "dyad" as a management model in integrated health systems. Physician Exec 2010;36:14–9.
6. Phillips RA, Cyr J, Keaney JF, et al. Creating and maintaining a successful service line in an academic medical center at the dawn of value-based care. Acad Med 2015;90:1340–6.

Important Quality Metrics and Standardization in Endoscopy

Tossapol Kerdsirichairat, MD[a], Eun Ji Shin, MD, PhD[b],*

KEYWORDS

- Quality metrics • Quality indicators • Standardization • Benchmarking
- Quality improvement • Endoscopy

KEY POINTS

- Following the Affordable Care Act of 2010, value-based reimbursement is emphasized, resulting in significant development of quality metrics and standardization in endoscopy.
- The Center for Medicare and Medicaid Services certifies the GI Quality Improvement Consortium registry as one of the methods for its Physician Quality Reporting Systems.
- Development and validation of quality measures, especially for ERCP and EUS, are required to meet the Affordable Care Act's triple aim of enhanced patient experience, better population health, and reduced costs.
- Quality metrics for endoscopy units in the era of COVID-19 are now developed as per the international Delphi consensus. The validation and data to show that the consensus improves the safety of patients and healthcare professionals are anticipated.

INTRODUCTION

The Institute of Medicine defines quality in health care as the degree to which healthcare services for individuals and populations increase the likelihood of desired health outcomes and are consistent with current professional knowledge.[1,2] Quality improvement consists of systematic and continuous actions that lead to measurable improvement in services. Processes related to quality improvement were initiated in 1959 at the Tokyo Institute of Technology. Processes consist of four steps including "plan–do–check–act".[3,4] This has been further refined to a process called Six Sigma, which was first implemented at Motorola in 1986 and at General Electric in 1995. This term derived from the statistical modeling of the manufacturing processes in which 99.9996% of all opportunities are statistically expected to be free of defects.[5,6] There are two models

[a] Digestive Disease Center, Bumrungrad International Hospital, Bangkok, Thailand 33 Soi Sukhumvit 3, Wattana, Bangkok 10110 Thailand; [b] Division of Gastroenterology and Hepatology, Department of Medicine, Johns Hopkins Medical Institutions, 1800 Orleans Street, Sheikh Zayed Tower, Suite 7125H, Baltimore, MD 21287, USA
* Corresponding author.
E-mail address: eshin3@jhmi.edu

Gastrointest Endoscopy Clin N Am 31 (2021) 727–742
https://doi.org/10.1016/j.giec.2021.05.009
1052-5157/21/© 2021 Elsevier Inc. All rights reserved.

of Six Sigma including DMAIC (define, measure, analyze, improve, control) and DMADV (define, measure, analyze, design, verify). It has been widely used in the fields of manufacturing, engineering and construction, finance, supply chain, and healthcare. In the field of healthcare, it was further modified using a lean Six Sigma.[7]

Approximately 44,000 to 98,000 Americans suffer and die from medical errors annually.[8] Therefore, the Institute of Medicine has developed 3 domains of quality control including safety, practice consistency, and customization, and implemented these quality measurements for performance evaluations to reimbursement.[8] Additional data have also confirmed that quality improvement in the healthcare system was associated with improved adherence to societal guidelines, cost-effectiveness, cost savings, improved quality of life, and improved survival.[9–11] Therefore, the models based on value-based care have become a standard of care for reimbursement, punishments, and credentialing.[12–15] The quality metrics related to disinfection, endoscope reprocessing, and quality control of anesthesia in endoscopy are included in other parts of this volume.

COMPONENTS AND DEFINITIONS IN QUALITY IMPROVEMENT

To perform quality improvement, multiple quality metrics have been developed in the form of structural measures, process measures, and outcomes measures.[16] Structural measures evaluate the system's capacity to provide care and might include the number of hospital beds, type of electronic medical records, or physician-to-patient ratio. Process measures evaluate processes of care, such as the proportion of patients vaccinated, and emergency room wait times.[17] Competency, defined as the minimum level of skill, knowledge, and experience required to safely and proficiently perform a task or procedure, is part of the structural measures and process measures. The criteria of competency can be varied depending on specialty, subspecialty, indications, types of procedure, and geographic locations.[18–22] Multiple studies have attempted to identify and validate the minimal procedure number, as well as evaluate the educational background and learning skills, to be able to provide credentialing and privileging.[18–24] Credentialing is the process in which an institution reviews an endoscopist's qualification to determine if they meet the criteria to perform the endoscopy procedure in question. The hospital credentialing committee will grant privileges based on the supporting evidence.[23,24] Outcome measures evaluate the outcomes of care and might include measures such as death from coronary syndrome, and the number of pressure ulcers in an assisted living facility.[17] An appropriate ratio of these 3 components will be calculated and reported in the form of a scorecard so that it can be compared among institutions.

Once the quality metrics are measured, the next step is to compare these metrics to the set standards. This step is called benchmarking, which can be further classified into internal benchmarking and external benchmarking. An example of internal benchmarking is comparing quality measures over a particular period among endoscopists in the same endoscopy unit. An example of external benchmarking is comparing the individual endoscopy unit quality metrics to the national societal standards.[25,26] Once variability in the performance of the metrics is identified during benchmarking, the step to implement the changes toward the set standards is standardization.

QUALITY METRICS FOR ENDOSCOPY UNITS

The first model in quality metrics for endoscopy units is the Global Rating Scale (GRS). This model is a web-based tool and further validated as a quality assessment tool for endoscopy services in the United Kingdom, Canada, and the Netherlands.[27–30] The GRS has 2 main dimensions: clinical quality and patient experience.[28] Clinical quality dimension consists of 6 domains including (1) information and consent, (2) safety, (3) processes that are in place to monitor patient comfort throughout the procedures, (4) quality assessment of procedure, (5) appropriateness of indications and policies for endoscopies, and (6) communication to the referrer. The patient experience dimension consists of 6 domains including (1) equality and equity for minority populations, (2) timeliness, (3) the planning of endoscopy programs and whether patients are given a choice in scheduling procedures, (4) privacy and dignity, (5) assessment of aftercare protocol such as discharge instructions and communication of results, and (6) ability for the patient to provide feedback.

The most commonly used quality metrics are based on that proposed by the American Society of Gastrointestinal Endoscopy (ASGE) to define high-quality endoscopy units (**Table 1**).[31] The taskforce consisted of gastroenterologists and nurses from various practice settings, both in the United States and internationally. The survey was performed using the Delphi method through 5 aspects including patient experience, employee experience, efficiency and operations, procedure-related endoscopy unit issues, and safety and infection control. There are 5 priority endoscopy unit quality indicators identified through this process including (1) a defined leadership structure, (2) regular education, training programs, and continuous quality improvement for all staff on new equipment/devices and endoscopic techniques, (3) endoscopy unit records, tracks, and monitors procedure quality indicators for both the endoscopy unit and individual endoscopists, (4) procedure reports are communicated to referring providers, and a process is in place for patients to receive a copy of the endoscopy report, and (5) a process is in place to track each specific endoscope from storage, use, reprocessing, and back to storage.[31]

In addition, the American College of Gastroenterology (ACG) along with the ASGE has proposed quality indicators common to all gastrointestinal endoscopy procedures.[32] The vast majority of the grade of recommendation was 3, defined as an unclear benefit, with expert opinion only, resulting in a weak recommendation and likely to be changed as data become available. Most quality indicators are classified as process measures. In general, priority quality indicators in the guidelines include (1) an appropriate and documented indication that is included in a published standard list, (2) use

Table 1
Guidelines related to quality indicators with a consensus using the Delphi method [a]

Types of Metrics	Organization(s)	Guidelines and Recommendations
Endoscopy units	ASGE	Quality indicators for GI endoscopy units[31]
	An international consensus	Recovery of endoscopy services in the area of COVID-19[109]
Preprocedural metrics	JGES	Guidelines for gastroenterological endoscopy in patients undergoing antithrombotic treatment
EGD	ACG-ASGE	Quality indicators for endoscopic eradication therapies in Barrett's esophagus
	JGES	Guidelines for endoscopic diagnosis of early gastric cancer[67]

Abbreviations: ACG, The American College of Gastroenterology; ASGE, the American Society of Gastrointestinal Endoscopy; EGD, esophagogastroduodenoscopy; JGES, the Japan Gastroenterological Endoscopy Society.
[a] Other guidelines proposed by societies without Delphi methods are not included in this table.

of prophylactic antibiotics for an appropriate indication, and (3) formulated and documented management of antithrombotic therapy before the procedure. More recently, the Korean Society of Gastrointestinal Endoscopy (KSGE) has proposed the criteria for an accredited endoscopy unit program in South Korea, with six categories including (1) qualification of endoscopists, (2) facilities and equipment, (3) process, (4) performance, (5) infection and infection control, and (6) sedation. Compared to the American guidelines, a unique mandatory item proposed by the KSGE is that each endoscopist must maintain at least 200 esophagogastroduodenoscopies (EGDs) and 100 colonoscopies every 3 years.[33]

QUALITY METRICS IN PROCEDURE-REPORTING SYSTEM

The European Society of Gastrointestinal Endoscopy (ESGE) quality improvement committee has proposed criteria in the reporting system in gastrointestinal endoscopy.[34] The methodology was based on expert opinion and was not performed using a Delphi process. Despite this limitation, it is recommended that the endoscopy reporting system (1) must be electronic, (2) should be integrated into hospital patient record systems, (3) should include patient identifiers to link to other data sources, (4) should restrict the use of free text entry, (5) should not have a separate entry of data for quality or research purposes, (6) should avoid double data entry by the endoscopist or associate personnel, (7) should include histopathology of detected lesions, patient satisfaction, adverse events, and surveillance recommendations, (8) can be retrieved at any time in a universally compatible format, (9) must include data fields for key performance indicators as defined by quality improvement committees, and (10) must facilitate changes in indicators and data entry fields as required by professional organizations.

Although there are no widely accepted protocol guidelines related to image documentation, the ESGE has suggested performing photodocumentation for at least 8 images for each of the upper endoscopy and colonoscopy. For upper endoscopy, the required images are (1) upper esophagus at 20 cm from the incisors, (2) lower esophagus at 2 cm above the squamocolumnar function, (3) gastric cardia in retroflexion view, (4) upper portion of the lesser curvature, (5) retroflection view of the angularis, (6) gastric antrum, (7) duodenal bulb, and (8) the second portion of the duodenum. In countries that have a higher prevalence of gastric cancer, a recommended time of examination remains similar to that of the USA, which is mostly 5 to 10 minutes. However, the Japanese endoscopists took more pictures (>20 pictures per EGD) compared to other Asian countries. Such practice has not been standardized or endorsed by societal guidelines.[35] The required photodocumentation for colonoscopy proposed by the ESGE includes (1) lower rectum, (2) middle portion of the sigmoid colon, (3) descending colon, (4) transverse colon adjacent to the splenic flexure, (5) transverse colon adjacent to the hepatic flexure, (6) ascending colon adjacent to the hepatic flexure, (7) ileocecal valve, and (8) cecum with visualization of the appendiceal orifice.[36] However, there are data showing that localization of the colon, especially in the left-sided colon, might not be accurate.[37–39] The subsequent ESGE guidelines did not emphasize the importance of photodocumenting the exact locations for colonoscopy.[34]

QUALITY METRICS FOR COLONOSCOPY

Compared to other types of endoscopic procedures, the development of quality metrics and standardization in the field of colonoscopy is most evidence-based and proven to be associated with improved patient outcomes. The most commonly used quality indicators for colonoscopy were proposed by the joint committees of the ACG/ASGE in 2015.[40,41] All of these indicators are classified as process measures and outcome measures. Preprocedural quality indicators include (1) documentation of appropriate indications, (2) fully documented informed consent, (3) indications based on guidelines for patients with postpolypectomy, postresection surveillance or average risks, and (4) documentation of specific intervals for those with inflammatory bowel disease. Intraprocedural quality indicators include (1) documentation of the quality of bowel prep, (2) documentation of whether the quality of bowel prep is adequate to allow the use of recommended surveillance or screening intervals, (3) photodocumentation of the cecum, (4) adenoma detection rate, (5) documentation of colonoscopy withdrawal time including 6 minutes or greater for screening colonoscopies with negative findings, (6) documentation of biopsies for an indication of chronic diarrhea, (7) documentation of tissue sampling for surveillance in inflammatory bowel disease, and (8) documentation of attempts to endoscopically remove a colonic polyp of smaller than 2 cm before surgical referral. Postprocedural quality indicators include (1) rate of perforation of less than 0.1% for screening colonoscopy, less than 0.2% for all other colonoscopies, and rate of postpolypectomy bleeding less than 1%, (2) greater than 90% of postpolypectomy bleeding should be managed without surgery, and (3) patients are provided with documentation for the timing of repeat colonoscopy.

Among these quality indicators, the ASGE/ACG has determined priority for colonoscopy indicators evaluating (1) adenoma detection rates ($\geq$30% in males and $\geq$20% in females) in asymptomatic average-risk individuals, (2) $\geq$90% colonoscopies follow recommended postpolypectomy and postcancer resection intervals and 10-year intervals screening colonoscopies in patients who have negative examination results and adequate bowel cleansing (performance target 90% or greater), and (3) visualization of the cecum ($\geq$90% for all examinations and $\geq$95% for screening) by notation of landmarks and photodocumentation of landmarks. The quality indicators will likely be further adjusted in the future based on several findings that (1) a second forward-view exam or a retroflexion of the right-sided colon improves adenoma detection rate,[42–48] and (2) requirements to collect and monitor report cards for each endoscopist.[49–51]

QUALITY METRICS FOR EGD

The joint committee of the ACG/ASGE has proposed quality indicators for EGD.[52,53] All of the indicators are classified as process measures. Preprocedural quality indicators include (1) documented indication as per a published standard list, (2) documented informed consent, (3) appropriate prophylactic antibiotics for patients with cirrhosis with acute upper GI bleeding before EGD, (4) appropriate antibiotics prior to placement of percutaneous endoscopic gastrostomy tube, (5) the use of proton pump inhibitor (PPI) suspected peptic ulcer bleeding, and (6) the use of vasoactive drugs before EGD for suspected variceal bleeding. Intraprocedural quality indicators include (1) complete examination and documentation of the esophagus, stomach including retroflection, and duodenum, (2) gastric biopsies for nonbleeding gastric ulcers to exclude malignancy, (3) accurate measurement in Barrett's esophagus, (4) esophageal biopsies for suspected Barrett's esophagus, (5) adequate description of types and locations of lesions, (6) adequate description of peptic ulcer, (7) appropriate treatment for ulcers with active bleeding or with nonbleeding visible vessels, (8) rates of achievement of primary hemostasis of documented bleeding lesions, (9) rates of secondary endoscopic modality performed when epinephrine is used as primary therapy for bleeding peptic ulcers, (10) rates of variceal ligation as primary therapy for esophageal varices, and (11) adequate intestinal biopsies for suspected celiac disease. Postprocedural quality metrics include (1) use of PPI after dilation for peptic esophageal strictures, (2) use of PPI or H2 antagonist in patients with gastric or duodenal ulcers, (3) plans to test for *Helicobacter pylori* infection for gastric or duodenal ulcers, (4) plan to perform a second look in patients with evidence of rebleeding from peptic ulcer, and (5) documentation that patients are contacted to monitor adverse events. Among these, the ACG/ASGE has prioritized 4 indicators including (1) greater than 98% of patients with ulcers with active bleeding or nonvisible vessel are treated endoscopically, (2) greater than 98% of patients with gastric or duodenal ulcers are with plans to test for *H pylori* infection, (3) greater than 98% of cirrhotic patients with acute upper GI bleeding receive appropriate prophylactic antibiotics before EGD, and (4) greater than 98% of patients with suspected peptic ulcer bleeding receive PPI.

Unlike the quality measures for colonoscopy, these quality measures for EGD have not been included in any value-based care plans, likely due to several factors including feasibility, detailed quality indicators, data burden to calculate metrics, and unintended consequences such that an extensive list of quality metrics may require resources to be diverted from other activities.[17] To simplify the current ACG/ASGE quality metrics for EGD, the newly proposed quality metrics for EGD are based on indications of the procedure. In Barrett's esophagus, the proposed metrics are (1) Barrett's inspection time can be used given that it is associated with increased detection of neoplasia, and (2) neoplasia detection rate as it can reflect adequate inspection of the Barrett segment.[54–58] In gastric cancer detection, the percentage of gastric intestinal metaplasia and gastric inspection time can be used.[57,59–61] The rate of proximal and distal esophageal biopsies for patients with suspected eosinophilic esophagitis is proposed as a quality metric.[62–66]

Recently, the Japanese Gastroenterological Endoscopy Society (JGES) developed a new guideline for early gastric cancer. In addition to the quality metrics proposed by the ACG/ASGE, the JGES suggested additional measures with either relatively strong strength of recommendation and/or level of evidence including (1) use of mucolytic agents to improve the visibility of gastric mucosa, (2) use of image-enhanced endoscopy to detect early gastric cancer and to evaluate the extent of invasion, (3) a close interval between screening EGD and therapeutic endoscopy procedures in the case of early gastric cancer, and (4) a surveillance EGD in patients with clinical and endoscopic risk factors for gastric cancers.[67]

QUALITY METRICS FOR ENDOSCOPIC RETROGRADE CHOLANGIOPANCREATOGRAPHY (ERCP)

Similar to more commonly performed procedures such as EGD and colonoscopy, the ACG/ASGE has proposed a list of quality indicators for ERCP.[68,69] The vast majority of these metrics are classified as process measures and outcome measures. Preprocedural quality metrics include (1) documentation of an appropriate indication, (2) documentation of informed consent, (3) use of appropriate antibiotics for indicated settings, (4) an ERCP performed by an endoscopist who is fully trained and credentialed, and (5) a recorded volume of ERCPs performed per year per endoscopist. Intraprocedural quality metrics include (1) documentation of deep cannulation of the ducts of interest, (2) rates of deep cannulation of the ducts of interest in native papillae without surgically altered anatomy, (3) documented and measured fluoroscopy time and radiation dose, (4) rate of successfully extracted common bile duct stone smaller than 1 cm in patients with normal bile duct anatomy, and (5) rate of successful stent placement for biliary obstruction in patients with normal anatomy whose biliary obstruction is below the bifurcation. Postprocedural metrics include (1) a complete ERCP report with descriptions on specific techniques, accessories used, and all intended outcomes, (2) documentation of acute adverse events and hospital transfers, (3) rates of post-ERCP pancreatitis, (4) rate and type of perforation, (5) rate of clinically significant hemorrhage after sphincterotomy or sphincteroplasty, and (6) documentation that patients are contacted at 14 days or after to detect and record the occurrence of delayed adverse events after ERCP. The ACG/ASGE suggested priority for (1) a documented indication, (2) success rate of greater than 90% for each of deep cannulation in native papillae, successful retrieval of common bile duct stone smaller than 1 cm, and successful biliary stenting for obstruction lower than the bifurcation, and (3) rate of post-ERCP pancreatitis. It should be noted that the task force did not provide the performance target for the rate of post-ERCP pancreatitis. The requirement of documentation regarding types of periprocedural prophylaxis of post-ERCP pancreatitis has been proposed by the ESGE.[70] The algorithm is based on whether pancreatic duct cannulation is encountered, and whether a patient has any contraindication to rectal nonsteroidal antiinflammatory drugs or high-volume intravenous lactated Ringer's solution. In general, the ESGE recommends routine rectal administration of 100 mg of diclofenac or indomethacin immediately before ERCP in all patients without contraindications.

QUALITY METRICS FOR ENDOSCOPIC ULTRASONOGRAPHY (EUS)

The ACG/ASGE taskforce has proposed quality indicators for EUS.[71,72] Preprocedural quality metrics include (1) documentation of appropriate indications, (2) documentation of informed consent, (3) use of appropriate antibiotics in the setting of fine-needle aspiration (FNA) of cystic lesions, and (4) EUS exams are performed by trained endosonographers. It should be noted that a recent randomized control trial showed that antibiotic prophylaxis is not required for FNA of pancreatic cystic lesions and such quality metric might be adjusted in the future.[73] Intraprocedural quality metrics include (1) documentation of the appearance of the structures specific to the indication for the EUS, (2) all gastrointestinal cancers are staged using the American Joint Committee on Cancer (AJCC)/Union for International Cancer Control TNM staging system, (3) documentation of vascular involvement, lymphadenopathy, distant metastasis in the setting of pancreatic masses including its measurement, (4) documentation of wall layers involved by a subepithelial lesion, (5) a tissue sampling of the primary tumor and lesions outside the primary field such as distant metastasis, ascites, and lymphadenopathy when it would alter patient management, (6) adequate sampling in all solid lesions, and (7) diagnostic rate and sensitivity of malignancy in patients with pancreatic mass. Postprocedural quality metrics include (1) documentation and limited incidence of adverse events after FNA such as pancreatitis, bleeding, perforation, and infection. The task force proposed priority quality indicators as follows: documentation of all GI cancers being staged using the AJCC TNM system (>98%), diagnostic rate and sensitivity for malignancy in patients with a pancreatic mass of greater than 70% and greater than 85%, respectively, rates of acute pancreatitis, perforation, and clinically significant bleeding of less than 2%, less than 0.5%, and less than 1%, respectively.

QUALITY METRICS FOR TRAINING ENDOSCOPY AND CREDENTIALING

Traditionally, the ACG/ASGE has suggested thresholds for competency of at a minimum 130 EGDs, 200 colonoscopies, 25 to 30 flexible sigmoidoscopies, 180 to 200 ERCPs, and 100 EUSs, while the American College of Surgeons requires 50 colonoscopies and 35 EGDs to be able to graduate from general surgery residency.[18,74–77] Based on the current training in EGD and colonoscopy, all third-year trainees of the academic year 2016 to 2017 who were prospectively evaluated throughout their fellowship training can achieve competence, validating the effectiveness of the current training programs in the USA.[78] This correlates with the data from the United Kingdom showing that credentialing was awarded after a median of 265 colonoscopies over 3.1 years.[79] However, recent data showed that advanced endoscopy trainees achieved competence in core EUS and ERCP skills at approximately 225 and 250 cases, respectively, and a higher grade of ERCP competence can be achieved at about 300 cases.[77,80] These documented numbers of EUSs and ERCPs performed during training can be used as a preprocedural quality measure instead of a broad assertion of a fully trained and credentialed endoscopist competent to perform EUS and ERCP.

BENCHMARKING AND STANDARDIZATION IN ENDOSCOPY

Once the endoscopy unit can internally measure and externally compare quality metrics against standards, quality assurance and quality improvement programs should be pursued.[26] Such steps become more critical because of the Patient Protection and Affordable Care Act of 2010.[81,82] Prior to the Medicare Access and Children's Health Insurance Program (CHIP) Reauthorization Act (MACRA), there were 8 basic methods of payment used as healthcare reimbursement, and all were related to the volume of the services.[83–85] The ACA has the goal of the triple aim of enhanced patient experience, better population health, and reduced costs.[86,87] This has shifted the reimbursement system from volume-based to value-based payment structure.[88,89] Starting in 2019, MACRA mandates that payments will completely fall through one of the two pathways chosen by the practice upfront.[90–93] The first pathway, the Merit-based Incentive Payment System (MIPS), combines traditional Medicare incentive programs (Meaningful Use and Physicians Quality Reporting Systems [PQRS]) with an individualized Quality and Resource Use Report, reflecting how much a practitioner spends on caring for Medicare patients. Medicare will derive a value-based modifier that will be applied to Medicare Part B payments. The second pathway is the alternative payment model that will grant an annual bonus of up to 5% of the prior year's Part B payments, but places on the practice an increased financial risk and greater demand for clinical integration. Therefore, quality metrics, benchmarking, and standardization are the backbone for this value-based payment structure, such that the US Centers for Medicare and Medicaid Services (CMS) requires 5 components including (1) an indication of age-appropriate screening colonoscopy, (2) appropriate follow-up interval after a normal colonoscopy in an average-risk patient, (3) appropriate colonoscopy intervals with a history of adenomatous polyps, (4) adenoma detection rates, and (5) photodocumentation of cecal intubation.[94,95] There are 3 pathways to capture, report, benchmark, and standardize quality in endoscopy to serve data to CMS.

The first pathway is through clinical data registries. This is traditionally used for research and quality reporting as it could avoid biases. It requires active participation to enter the data from multiple sources, which can be time-consuming and costly. The most commonly used, based on this pathway, is the GI quality improvement consortium (GIQuIC) proposed by the ASGE/ACG.[96,97] GIQuIC is currently limited to EGD and colonoscopy, and is expected to expand to ERCP.[98] The American Gastroenterological Association (AGA) Digestive Health Outcomes Registry and GIQuIC are the only 2 methods for an official PQRS registry.[82] The second pathway is claims-based administrative data from insurance companies, billing records, and national databases. This pathway has several advantages including its readily available data with a large sample size, identification of health disparities, and the dynamics of reimbursement over time.[94] However, it lacks clinical outcomes, final pathology, and/or adverse events. In addition, the coding does not often reflect the quality measurement.[99] The third pathway is the electronic health record (EHR)-based measurement that can capture clinically accurate and readily available data in a more real-time manner.[94,95] The disadvantages of this pathway are (1) inconsistent and missing terminology and documentation, (2) transferability of different EHR systems, (3) lack of standardized data structure, and (4) requirements of additional steps to use as an official PQRS registry. Once natural language processing is fully developed, this pathway might be ideal, as demonstrated by the Veterans Affairs EHR-dependent quality measurement to identify overuse of screening colonoscopy.[100–105]

QUALITY METRICS IN THE ERA OF COVID-19

There are many recommendations proposed by societies regarding quality metrics during the time of the pandemic, proposed by the AGA, the ASGE, the Asia-Pacific Society for Digestive Endoscopy, the British Society of Gastroenterology, and the Digestive Health Physicians Association, with consensus items including (1) preendoscopy clinical screening for all patients, (2) deferment of elective endoscopy patients with suspected or confirmed COVID-19, (3) in the absence of active testing, all patients should be presumed to be infective and healthcare professionals should wear enhanced personal protective equipment, (4) deep cleaning of the procedure room after every procedure, and (5) strict adherence to endoscope disinfection policies.[106–108] More recently, an international Delphi consensus was developed with additional specific recommendations. Additional and measurable preprocedural metrics include (1) all patients undergoing endoscopy procedures should be tested for SARS-CoV-2 infection 24 to 72 hours prior to endoscopy in high-prevalence regions, (2) point-of-care tests for detection of active infection could be used in high-prevalence regions, (3) in the absence of universal testing, patients receiving therapeutic endoscopy procedures lasting longer than 1 hour should be tested for SARS-CoV2 infection in high-prevalence regions, (4) all healthcare professionals working in endoscopy should be tested once for SARS-CoV-2 infection, undergo symptom-and-temperature checks, and regular retesting in high-prevalence regions considered, and (5) all patients attending for endoscopy procedures should wear simple surgical mask at all times apart from the time when an endoscope has to be inserted into the oral cavity, and all healthcare professionals should wear a surgical mask at all times in clinical areas. Additional and measurable intraprocedural metrics are (1) healthcare professionals using N95/FFP3 during upper and lower GI procedures in high-prevalence regions and a surgical mask during colonoscopy in low-prevalence regions, (2) donning and doffing areas should be separated and located outside endoscopy rooms, and (3) all suspected or confirmed COVID-19 infections should have an endoscopy in negative-pressure rooms. Additional and measurable postprocedural metrics are (1) the doffing area could be in one corner of the room, (2) the endoscopy room should be deep cleaned after every procedure in a suspected or confirmed COVID-19 case, (3) patients with suspected or confirmed COVID-19 should be recovering in an area away from all other non-COVID-19 patients, (4) in high-prevalence regions, healthcare professionals in the endoscopy recovery areas should wear standard personal protective equipment with surgical masks, and (5) all patients should be followed-up by phone in 10 to 14 days to identify any symptoms suggestive of COVID-19 in high-prevalence regions.[109]

AREAS OF RESEARCH OF QUALITY METRICS AND STANDARDIZATION IN ENDOSCOPY

A consensus using the Delphi method to identify appropriate reporting systems for endoscopic procedures other than colonoscopy that show improved patient outcomes should be developed and validated. More criteria on structural metrics and outcome metrics with validation of performance targets are required for most quality indicators for EGD, ERCP, and EUS. A comparative study using the GRS versus the ACG/ASGE quality metrics for endoscopy units with impacts on patient outcomes should be conducted. Quality metrics regarding photodocumentation other than the cecum should be conducted for other procedures. A comparative study of the ACG/ASGE versus the indication-based AGA guidelines should be performed to identify feasible and simplified quality metrics for EGD. Quality indicators for interventional EUS are awaiting. A study to show that base numbers required for EUS and ERCP credentialing can improve patient outcomes is required. Lastly, quality metrics for reopening or continuing endoscopy units in low-prevalence regions (eg, Taiwan, Thailand, and New Zealand), especially in the setting of ongoing trials of a vaccine against SARS-CoV-2, are necessary.[110]

CLINICS CARE POINTS

1. Endoscopy units are encouraged to follow the American Society of Gastrointestinal Endoscopy (ASGE) guidelines to be qualified as high-quality endoscopy units and the Asian Pacific Society for Digestive Endoscopy recommendations in the era of COVID-19.

2. Most important quality metrics for colonoscopy include adenoma detection rate, appropriate recommendation of interval colonoscopy, and visualization of the cecum.

3. Quality metrics in upper endoscopy are mainly based on Barrett's esophagus (inspection time and neoplasia detection rate) and gastric cancer detection (gastric inspection time and rate of gastric intestinal metaplasia detection).

4. Routine rectal indomethacin should be implemented in all patients undergoing ERCPs without contraindications.

DISCLOSURE

T. Kerdsirichairat declares no conflict of interest. E.J. Shin, MD PhD has served as a consultant for Boston Scientific, United States and received a research grant from Augmenix, Inc., United States.

REFERENCES

1. Kohn L. To err is human: an interview with the Institute of Medicine's Linda Kohn. Jt Comm J Qual Improv 2000;26:227–34.
2. Havens DH, Boroughs L. "To err is human": a report from the Institute of Medicine. J Pediatr Health Care 2000;14:77–80.
3. Nicolay CR, Purkayastha S, Greenhalgh A, et al. Systematic review of the application of quality improvement methodologies from the manufacturing industry to surgical healthcare. Br J Surg 2012;99:324–35.
4. Hill JE, Stephani AM, Sapple P, et al. The effectiveness of continuous quality improvement for developing professional practice and improving health care outcomes: a systematic review. Implement Sci 2020;15:23.

5. Ninerola A, Sanchez-Rebull MV, Hernandez-Lara AB. Quality improvement in healthcare: Six Sigma systematic review. Health Policy 2020;124:438–45.
6. Gras JM, Philippe M. Application of the Six Sigma concept in clinical laboratories: a review. Clin Chem Lab Med 2007;45:789–96.
7. de Koning H, Verver JP, van den Heuvel J, et al. Lean six sigma in healthcare. J Healthc Qual 2006;28:4–11.
8. Kohn LT, Corrigan JM, Donaldson MS, editors. To err is human: building a safer health system. 2000. Washington (DC).
9. Johnson EA, Spier BJ, Leff JA, et al. Optimising the care of patients with cirrhosis and gastrointestinal haemorrhage: a quality improvement study. Aliment Pharmacol Ther 2011;34:76–82.
10. Tapper EB, Friderici J, Borman ZA, et al. A multicenter evaluation of adherence to 4 major elements of the Baveno guidelines and outcomes for patients with acute variceal hemorrhage. J Clin Gastroenterol 2018;52:172–7.
11. Kennedy NA, Rodgers A, Altus R, et al. Optimisation of hepatocellular carcinoma surveillance in patients with viral hepatitis: a quality improvement study. Intern Med J 2013;43:772–7.
12. Baker DW, Yendro S. Setting achievable benchmarks for value-based payments: no perfect solution. JAMA 2018;319:1857–8.
13. Roberts ET, Zaslavsky AM, McWilliams JM. The value-based payment modifier: program outcomes and implications for disparities. Ann Intern Med 2018;168: 255–65.
14. Chen LM, Epstein AM, Orav EJ, et al. Association of practice-level social and medical risk with performance in the Medicare physician value-based payment modifier program. JAMA 2017;318:453–61.
15. Hirsch JA, Rosenkrantz AB, Ansari SA, et al. MACRA 2.0: are you ready for MIPS? J Neurointerv Surg 2017;9:714–6.
16. Kessell E, Pegany V, Keolanui B, et al. Review of Medicare, Medicaid, and commercial quality of care measures: considerations for assessing accountable care organizations. J Health Polit Policy Law 2015;40:761–96.
17. Sharma P, Parasa S, Shaheen N. Developing quality metrics for upper endoscopy. Gastroenterology 2020;158:9–13.
18. Jowell PS, Baillie J, Branch MS, et al. Quantitative assessment of procedural competence. A prospective study of training in endoscopic retrograde cholangiopancreatography. Ann Intern Med 1996;125:983–9.
19. Verma D, Gostout CJ, Petersen BT, et al. Establishing a true assessment of endoscopic competence in ERCP during training and beyond: a single-operator learning curve for deep biliary cannulation in patients with native papillary anatomy. Gastrointest Endosc 2007;65:394–400.
20. Shahidi N, Ou G, Telford J, et al. When trainees reach competency in performing ERCP: a systematic review. Gastrointest Endosc 2015;81:1337–42.
21. Siau K, Crossley J, Dunckley P, et al. Colonoscopy direct observation of procedural skills assessment tool for evaluating competency development during training. Am J Gastroenterol 2020;115:234–43.
22. Miller AT, Sedlack RE, Group ACER. Competency in esophagogastroduodenoscopy: a validated tool for assessment and generalizable benchmarks for gastroenterology fellows. Gastrointest Endosc 2019;90:613–620 e1.
23. Yang D, Wagh MS, Draganov PV. The status of training in new technologies in advanced endoscopy: from defining competence to credentialing and privileging. Gastrointest Endosc 2020;92:1016–25.

24. Eisen GM, Baron TH, Dominitz JA, et al. Methods of granting hospital privileges to perform gastrointestinal endoscopy. Gastrointest Endosc 2002;55:780–3.

25. Morris EJ, Rutter MD, Finan PJ, et al. Post-colonoscopy colorectal cancer (PCCRC) rates vary considerably depending on the method used to calculate them: a retrospective observational population-based study of PCCRC in the English National Health Service. Gut 2015;64:1248–56.

26. Petersen BT. Quality assurance for endoscopists. Best Pract Res Clin Gastroenterol 2011;25:349–60.

27. Williams T, Ross A, Stirling C, et al. Validation of the Global Rating Scale for endoscopy. Scott Med J 2013;58:20–1.

28. Sint Nicolaas J, de Jonge V, de Man RA, et al. The Global Rating Scale in clinical practice: a comprehensive quality assurance programme for endoscopy departments. Dig Liver Dis 2012;44:919–24.

29. Sint Nicolaas J, de Jonge V, Korfage IJ, et al. Benchmarking patient experiences in colonoscopy using the Global Rating Scale. Endoscopy 2012;44:462–72.

30. MacIntosh D, Dube C, Hollingworth R, et al. The endoscopy Global Rating Scale-Canada: development and implementation of a quality improvement tool. Can J Gastroenterol 2013;27:74–82.

31. Taskforce AEUQI, Day LW, Cohen J, et al. Quality indicators for gastrointestinal endoscopy units. VideoGIE 2017;2:119–40.

32. Rizk MK, Sawhney MS, Cohen J, et al. Quality indicators common to all GI endoscopic procedures. Am J Gastroenterol 2015;110:48–59.

33. Kim JW, Cho YK, Kim JO, et al. Accredited endoscopy unit program of Korea: overview and qualification. Clin Endosc 2019;52:426–30.

34. Bretthauer M, Aabakken L, Dekker E, et al. Reporting systems in gastrointestinal endoscopy: Requirements and standards facilitating quality improvement: European Society of Gastrointestinal Endoscopy position statement. United Eur Gastroenterol J 2016;4:172–6.

35. Uedo N, Gotoda T, Yoshinaga S, et al. Differences in routine esophagogastroduodenoscopy between Japanese and international facilities: A questionnaire survey. Dig Endosc 2016;28(Suppl 1):16–24.

36. Rey JF, Lambert R, Committee EQA. ESGE recommendations for quality control in gastrointestinal endoscopy: guidelines for image documentation in upper and lower GI endoscopy. Endoscopy 2001;33:901–3.

37. Vaziri K, Choxi SC, Orkin BA. Accuracy of colonoscopic localization. Surg Endosc 2010;24:2502–5.

38. Nayor J, Rotman SR, Chan WW, et al. Endoscopic localization of colon cancer is frequently inaccurate. Dig Dis Sci 2017;62:2120–5.

39. Fernandez LM, Ibrahim RNM, Mizrahi I, et al. How accurate is preoperative colonoscopic localization of colonic neoplasia? Surg Endosc 2019;33:1174–9.

40. Rex DK, Schoenfeld PS, Cohen J, et al. Quality indicators for colonoscopy. Gastrointest Endosc 2015;81:31–53.

41. Rex DK, Schoenfeld PS, Cohen J, et al. Quality indicators for colonoscopy. Am J Gastroenterol 2015;110:72–90.

42. Tang RSY, Lee JWJ, Chang LC, et al. Two vs one forward view examination of right colon on adenoma detection: an international multicenter randomized trial. Clin Gastroenterol Hepatol 2020. https://doi.org/10.1016/j.cgh.2020.10.014.

43. Desai M, Bilal M, Hamade N, et al. Increasing adenoma detection rates in the right side of the colon comparing retroflexion with a second forward view: a systematic review. Gastrointest Endosc 2019;89:453–459 e3.

44. Chandran S, Parker F, Vaughan R, et al. Right-sided adenoma detection with retroflexion versus forward-view colonoscopy. Gastrointest Endosc 2015;81: 608–13.

45. Hewett DG, Rex DK. Miss rate of right-sided colon examination during colonoscopy defined by retroflexion: an observational study. Gastrointest Endosc 2011; 74:246–52.

46. Cohen J, Grunwald D, Grossberg LB, et al. The effect of right colon retroflexion on adenoma detection: a systematic review and meta-analysis. J Clin Gastroenterol 2017;51:818–24.

47. Clark BT, Parikh ND, Laine L. Yield of repeat forward-view examination of the right side of the colon in screening and surveillance colonoscopy. Gastrointest Endosc 2016;84:126–32.

48. Kushnir VM, Oh YS, Hollander T, et al. Impact of retroflexion vs. second forward view examination of the right colon on adenoma detection: a comparison study. Am J Gastroenterol 2015;110:415–22.

49. Duloy AM, Kaltenbach TR, Wood M, et al. Colon polypectomy report card improves polypectomy competency: results of a prospective quality improvement study (with video). Gastrointest Endosc 2019;89:1212–21.

50. Keswani RN, Yadlapati R, Gleason KM, et al. Physician report cards and implementing standards of practice are both significantly associated with improved screening colonoscopy quality. Am J Gastroenterol 2015;110:1134–9.

51. Kahi CJ, Ballard D, Shah AS, et al. Impact of a quarterly report card on colonoscopy quality measures. Gastrointest Endosc 2013;77:925–31.

52. Park WG, Shaheen NJ, Cohen J, et al. Quality indicators for EGD. Gastrointest Endosc 2015;81:17–30.

53. Park WG, Shaheen NJ, Cohen J, et al. Quality indicators for EGD. Am J Gastroenterol 2015;110:60–71.

54. Desai M, Sharma P. What quality metrics should we apply in Barrett's esophagus? Am J Gastroenterol 2019;114:1197–8.

55. Falk GW. 2017 David Sun Lecture: Screening and surveillance of Barrett's esophagus: where are we now and what does the future hold? Am J Gastroenterol 2019;114:64–70.

56. Gupta N, Gaddam S, Wani SB, et al. Longer inspection time is associated with increased detection of high-grade dysplasia and esophageal adenocarcinoma in Barrett's esophagus. Gastrointest Endosc 2012;76:531–8.

57. Park JM, Huo SM, Lee HH, et al. Longer observation time increases proportion of neoplasms detected by esophagogastroduodenoscopy. Gastroenterology 2017;153:460–469 e1.

58. Parasa S, Desai M, Vittal A, et al. Estimating neoplasia detection rate (NDR) in patients with Barrett's oesophagus based on index endoscopy: a systematic review and meta-analysis. Gut 2019;68:2122–8.

59. Dinis-Ribeiro M, Areia M, de Vries AC, et al. Management of precancerous conditions and lesions in the stomach (MAPS): guideline from the European Society of Gastrointestinal Endoscopy (ESGE), European Helicobacter Study Group (EHSG), European Society of Pathology (ESP), and the Sociedade Portuguesa de Endoscopia Digestiva (SPED). Endoscopy 2012;44:74–94.

60. Pimentel-Nunes P, Libanio D, Marcos-Pinto R, et al. Management of epithelial precancerous conditions and lesions in the stomach (MAPS II): European Society of Gastrointestinal Endoscopy (ESGE), European Helicobacter and Microbiota Study Group (EHMSG), European Society of Pathology (ESP), and

Sociedade Portuguesa de Endoscopia Digestiva (SPED) guideline update 2019. Endoscopy 2019;51:365–88.

61. Teh JL, Tan JR, Lau LJ, et al. Longer examination time improves detection of gastric cancer during diagnostic upper gastrointestinal endoscopy. Clin Gastroenterol Hepatol 2015;13:480–7.e2.

62. Shah A, Kagalwalla AF, Gonsalves N, et al. Histopathologic variability in children with eosinophilic esophagitis. Am J Gastroenterol 2009;104:716–21.

63. Nielsen JA, Lager DJ, Lewin M, et al. The optimal number of biopsy fragments to establish a morphologic diagnosis of eosinophilic esophagitis. Am J Gastroenterol 2014;109:515–20.

64. Krarup AL, Drewes AM, Ejstrud P, et al. Implementation of a biopsy protocol to improve detection of esophageal eosinophilia: a Danish registry-based study. Endoscopy 2020;53:15–24.

65. Sperry SL, Shaheen NJ, Dellon ES. Toward uniformity in the diagnosis of eosinophilic esophagitis (EoE): the effect of guidelines on variability of diagnostic criteria for EoE. Am J Gastroenterol 2011;106:824–32 [quiz: 833].

66. Dellon ES, Aderoju A, Woosley JT, et al. Variability in diagnostic criteria for eosinophilic esophagitis: a systematic review. Am J Gastroenterol 2007;102:2300–13.

67. Yao K, Uedo N, Kamada T, et al. Guidelines for endoscopic diagnosis of early gastric cancer. Dig Endosc 2020;32:663–98.

68. Adler DG, Lieb JG 2nd, Cohen J, et al. Quality indicators for ERCP. Am J Gastroenterol 2015;110:91–101.

69. Adler DG, Lieb JG 2nd, Cohen J, et al. Quality indicators for ERCP. Gastrointest Endosc 2015;81:54–66.

70. Dumonceau JM, Kapral C, Aabakken L, et al. ERCP-related adverse events: European Society of Gastrointestinal Endoscopy (ESGE) Guideline. Endoscopy 2020;52:127–49.

71. Wani S, Wallace MB, Cohen J, et al. Quality indicators for EUS. Am J Gastroenterol 2015;110:102–13.

72. Wani S, Wallace MB, Cohen J, et al. Quality indicators for EUS. Gastrointest Endosc 2015;81:67–80.

73. Colan-Hernandez J, Sendino O, Loras C, et al. Antibiotic prophylaxis is not required for endoscopic ultrasonography-guided fine-needle aspiration of pancreatic cystic lesions, based on a randomized trial. Gastroenterology 2020;158:1642–9.e1.

74. Watkins JL, Etzkorn KP, Wiley TE, et al. Assessment of technical competence during ERCP training. Gastrointest Endosc 1996;44:411–5.

75. Cass OW, Freeman ML, Peine CJ, et al. Objective evaluation of endoscopy skills during training. Ann Intern Med 1993;118:40–4.

76. Han S, Obuch JC, Keswani RN, et al. Effect of individualized feedback on learning curves in EGD and colonoscopy: a cluster randomized controlled trial. Gastrointest Endosc 2020;91:882–93.e4.

77. Wani S, Han S, Simon V, et al. Setting minimum standards for training in EUS and ERCP: results from a prospective multicenter study evaluating learning curves and competence among advanced endoscopy trainees. Gastrointest Endosc 2019;89:1160–1168 e9.

78. Han S, Obuch JC, Duloy AM, et al. A prospective multicenter study evaluating endoscopy competence among gastroenterology trainees in the era of the next accreditation system. Acad Med 2020;95:283–92.

79. Siau K, Hodson J, Valori RM, et al. Performance indicators in colonoscopy after certification for independent practice: outcomes and predictors of competence. Gastrointest Endosc 2019;89:482–92.e2.
80. Wani S, Keswani RN, Han S, et al. Competence in endoscopic ultrasound and endoscopic retrograde cholangiopancreatography, from training through independent practice. Gastroenterology 2018;155:1483–94.e7.
81. Oberlander J. Learning from failure in health care reform. N Engl J Med 2007; 357:1677–9.
82. Allen JI. The road ahead. Clin Gastroenterol Hepatol 2012;10:692–6.
83. Golding LP, Nicola GN, Ansari SA, et al. MACRA 2.5: the legislation moves forward. J Neurointerv Surg 2018;10:1224–8.
84. Sommers BD, Musco T, Finegold K, et al. Health reform and changes in health insurance coverage in 2014. N Engl J Med 2014;371:867–74.
85. Quinn K. The 8 basic payment methods in health care. Ann Intern Med 2015; 163:300–6.
86. Berwick DM, Nolan TW, Whittington J. The triple aim: care, health, and cost. Health Aff (Millwood) 2008;27:759–69.
87. Allen JI. Gastroenterologists and the triple aim: how to become accountable. Gastrointest Endosc Clin N Am 2012;22:85–96.
88. Lopez MH, Daniel GW, Fiore NC, et al. Paying for value from costly medical technologies: a framework for applying value-based payment reforms. Health Aff (Millwood) 2020;39:1018–25.
89. Mayes R. Moving (realistically) from volume-based to value-based health care payment in the USA: starting with medicare payment policy. J Health Serv Res Policy 2011;16:249–51.
90. Centers for M, Medicaid Services HHS. Medicare Program; Merit-Based Incentive Payment System (MIPS) and Alternative Payment Model (APM) incentive under the physician fee schedule, and criteria for physician-focused payment models. Final rule with comment period. Fed Regist 2016;81:77008–831.
91. Jones RT, Helm B, Parris D, et al. The Medicare Access and CHIP Reauthorization Act of 2015 (MACRA) made simple for medical and radiation oncologists: a narrative review. JAMA Oncol 2019;5:723–7.
92. Brill JV, Jain R, Margolis PS, et al. A bundled payment framework for colonoscopy performed for colorectal cancer screening or surveillance. Gastroenterology 2014;146:849–53.e9.
93. Lieberman D, Allen J. New approaches to controlling health care costs: bending the cost curve for colonoscopy. JAMA Intern Med 2015;175:1789–91.
94. Adams MA, Saini SD, Allen JI. Quality measures in gastrointestinal endoscopy: the current state. Curr Opin Gastroenterol 2017;33:352–7.
95. Calderwood AH, Jacobson BC. Colonoscopy quality: metrics and implementation. Gastroenterol Clin North Am 2013;42:599–618.
96. Wani S, Williams JL, Falk GW, et al. An analysis of the GIQuIC nationwide quality registry reveals unnecessary surveillance endoscopies in patients with normal and irregular Z-lines. Am J Gastroenterol 2020;115:1869–78.
97. Shaukat A, Holub J, Greenwald D, et al. Variation over time and factors associated with detection rates of sessile serrated lesion across the United States: results form a national sample using the GIQuIC registry. Am J Gastroenterol 2020. https://doi.org/10.14309/ajg.0000000000000824.
98. Cotton PB. ERCP (Ensuring Really Competent Practice): enough words-action please! Gastrointest Endosc 2015;81:1343–5.

99. Williams JE, Holub JL, Faigel DO. Polypectomy rate is a valid quality measure for colonoscopy: results from a national endoscopy database. Gastrointest Endosc 2012;75:576–82.

100. Saini SD, Powell AA, Dominitz JA, et al. Developing and testing an electronic measure of screening colonoscopy overuse in a large integrated healthcare system. J Gen Intern Med 2016;31(Suppl 1):53–60.

101. Laique SN, Hayat U, Sarvepalli S, et al. Application of optical character recognition with natural language processing for large-scale quality metric data extraction in colonoscopy reports. Gastrointest Endosc 2020. https://doi.org/10.1016/j.gie.2020.08.038.

102. Imler TD, Sherman S, Imperiale TF, et al. Provider-specific quality measurement for ERCP using natural language processing. Gastrointest Endosc 2018;87:164–73.e2.

103. Raju GS, Lum PJ, Slack RS, et al. Natural language processing as an alternative to manual reporting of colonoscopy quality metrics. Gastrointest Endosc 2015;82:512–9.

104. Imler TD, Morea J, Kahi C, et al. Multi-center colonoscopy quality measurement utilizing natural language processing. Am J Gastroenterol 2015;110:543–52.

105. Gawron AJ, Thompson WK, Keswani RN, et al. Anatomic and advanced adenoma detection rates as quality metrics determined via natural language processing. Am J Gastroenterol 2014;109:1844–9.

106. Gralnek IM, Hassan C, Beilenhoff U, et al. ESGE and ESGENA position statement on gastrointestinal endoscopy and the COVID-19 pandemic. Endoscopy 2020;52:483–90.

107. Hennessy B, Vicari J, Bernstein B, et al. Guidance for resuming GI endoscopy and practice operations after the COVID-19 pandemic. Gastrointest Endosc 2020;92:743–747 e1.

108. Chiu PWY, Ng SC, Inoue H, et al. Practice of endoscopy during COVID-19 pandemic: position statements of the Asian Pacific Society for Digestive Endoscopy (APSDE-COVID statements). Gut 2020;69:991–6.

109. Bhandari P, Subramaniam S, Bourke MJ, et al. Recovery of endoscopy services in the era of COVID-19: recommendations from an international Delphi consensus. Gut 2020;69:1915–24.

110. The Centers for Disease Control and Prevention. COVID-19 travel recommendations by destination. Available at: https://www.cdc.gov/coronavirus/2019-ncov/travelers/map-and-travel-notices.html. Accessed November 11, 2020.

Adoption of New Technologies
Artificial Intelligence

Jeremy R. Glissen Brown, MD*, Tyler M. Berzin, MD, MS, FASGE

KEYWORDS

- Deep learning • Machine learning • Computer-aided detection
- Computer-aided diagnosis • Polyp detection • Operations • Cost-effectiveness
- Regulations

KEY POINTS

- Evidence is mounting for 2 broad areas of application in regards to artificial intelligence (AI) as applied to gastroenterology: computer-aided detection (CADe) and computer-aided diagnosis (CADx).
- Several prospective, randomized clinical trials support the use of CADe for the automatic detection of polyps in the colon. As these technologies are introduced to the endoscopy suite, the physician should become familiar with ways to incorporate AI technology in gastrointestinal endoscopy.
- Recent evidence suggests that in the future, CADx technology may support a "diagnose and leave" strategy for diminutive polyps in the rectosigmoid colon, obviating the need for polypectomy.
- AI also has the potential to optimize workflow in clinical encounters and in the endoscopy suite. Potential applications include using natural language processing to compile health records, optimize clinical note taking, and automatically generate endoscopy reports; using AI to improve endoscopy quality of care; and using machine learning techniques to generate prediction models that may be integrated into the electronic medical record in the future for clinical care.
- As CADe and CADx technologies continue to evolve and grow, there is a parallel need for regulatory pathways to evolve and directly address unique challenges that come with applying AI to clinical care. In addition, the cost-effectiveness of any intervention will need to be addressed.

Center for Advanced Endoscopy, Division of Gastroenterology and Hepatology, Beth Israel Deaconess Medical Center and Harvard Medical School, 330 Brookline Avenue, Boston, MA 02130, USA
* Corresponding author.
E-mail address: jglissen@bidmc.harvard.edu

Gastrointest Endoscopy Clin N Am 31 (2021) 743–758
https://doi.org/10.1016/j.giec.2021.05.010
1052-5157/21/© 2021 Elsevier Inc. All rights reserved.

INTRODUCTION

Over the past decade, artificial intelligence (AI) has captured the popular imagination. With advancements in computing power, the development of optimization algorithms, and the overall refinement of machine learning (ML) techniques, we have recently seen AI and ML applied to nearly every aspect of human life, with recent groundbreaking successes in facial recognition, natural language processing, autonomous driving, and medical imaging. In medicine, deep learning has been applied to a diverse array of clinical problems, from the detection of breast cancer on standard mammogram to the diagnosis of cutaneous malignancy and diabetic retinopathy.[1–3]

The field of gastroenterology has applied AI to a vast array of clinical problems, and some of the earliest prospective trials examining AI in medicine have been in computer vision applied to endoscopy.[4] Since that time, we have seen AI and ML applied to nearly every conceivable niche within gastroenterology.

As the field of AI within gastroenterology continues to mature and grow, it is important for gastroenterologists, key stakeholders in the conversation, to familiarize themselves with the technology, the common language, and the literature surrounding AI/ML in gastroenterology and gastrointestinal (GI) endoscopy.

In this article, the authors review basic terminology and then evidence for the broad subfield of *computer-aided detection* (*CADe*) as applied to gastroenterology, practical considerations when using CADe technology in the endoscopy suite, evidence for and applications of *computer-aided diagnosis* (*CADx*), and then future applications of AI/ML and important considerations from an operations standpoint.

DEFINITIONS AND TERMINOLOGY

Because the emerging field is one that combines work from clinicians, computer scientists, engineers, commercial entities, regulatory bodies, and patients, it is imperative that relevant stakeholders familiarize themselves with common terminology (**Table 1**). *Artificial Intelligence* is a branch of computer science dedicated to the creation of systems designed to perform tasks that classically require human intelligence. *Machine learning* is a set of computational methods that involves using mathematical models to learn to capture structure in data. This usually involves *training* on example data followed by *validation* and *testing* on a different data set in order to form predictions on unseen data.[5] *Deep learning* is a subset of ML that involves the extraction of many feature layers from raw data and that uses neural networks, which have been likened to the animal nervous system, to produce complex predictive outputs.[6] *Computer-aided detection* (*CADe*) involves the use of ML or deep learning for lesion detection, such as in the detection of polyps during colonoscopy. *Computer-aided diagnosis* (*CADx*) involves the use of ML or deep learning to predict diagnosis, such as in predicting malignant versus nonmalignant histology for colon polyps. *Training* involves using input data, often represented by *features* (for example, in the case of a CADe algorithm for the detection of polyps in the colon, edge, color, and texture features expressed numerically) to build a mathematical model and generate a prediction. With conventional ML methods, features are manually selected by researchers based on knowledge of the field, whereas in deep learning, the algorithm learns the best features from the data itself. Most current applications of ML within gastroenterology are examples of *supervised learning*, whereby input data are labeled (for example, by having expert endoscopists manually label images of polyps).

Table 1
Overview of commonly used terminology in machine learning

Machine learning	The use of mathematical models for capturing structure in data. After optimization on example data, so-called training, the models can be used to make predictions about new, unseen data
Features	Visual properties of the data that are quantitatively summarized in an array of numbers. In conventional machine learning, these features are clinically inspired and thus handcrafted, whereas in deep learning these features are automatically learned from the data
Computer-aided detection (CADe)	Machine learning algorithms applied to medical data for primary detection of pathologic condition (eg, polyp detection)
Computer-aided diagnosis (CADx)	Machine learning algorithms applied to medical data for predicting diagnoses (eg, polyp classification)
Deep learning	A form of machine learning in which a neural network of several layers is used, exploiting hierarchical relations in the data. The major difference from conventional machine learning is that these features and relations are all learned from the data, a property which is also referred to as end-to-end learning
Pretraining	Training a deep learning algorithm with data that are different from the target data. This technique can be exploited to first train a rough model on a large set that can be fine-tuned using a smaller data set of interest. ImageNet is the most commonly used data set for pretraining
Transfer learning	This is used after a deep neural network is pretrained on a large data set that is different from the target data. Generally, a data set is used with general imagery not specific to the final purpose of the algorithm. This pretrained model extracts basic discriminating features from the large data set, and these features and their weights are then "transferred" for training and fine-tuning on new data, which are specific to the target purpose of the new model.

(*Adapted from* van der Sommen F, de Groof J, Struyvenberg M et al. Machine learning in GI endoscopy: practical guidance in how to interpret a novel field. Gut. 2020 Nov;69(11):2035-2045.)

COMPUTER-AIDED DETECTION
History and Evidence: Computer-Aided Detection

In gastroenterology, the most mature application of ML and deep learning is CADe during colonoscopy and endoscopy. Early efforts involved creating polyp detection algorithms for use during colonoscopy using manual feature extraction methods on still images and then validation in retrospective video analysis.[7–9] Advances in deep learning have allowed for the development of more sophisticated, multilayer algorithms based on neural networks that are able to perform in near real-time with little or no detectable latency.[10]

In 2019, Wang and colleagues[4] published the first prospective, randomized clinical trial involving AI in medicine. This involved randomization of 1058 patients in a single endoscopy center in China to receive colonoscopy with or without the assistance of a CADe algorithm projected on a second endoscopy monitor. The investigators found a significant increase in adenoma detection rate (ADR) with an increase from 20.3% in the control arm to 29.1% in the experimental arm (odds ratio, 1.61; 95% confidence interval [CI], 1.213 to 2.135; $P<.001$) as well as an increase in the mean number of adenomas per colonoscopy. This was due to a higher number of diminutive adenomas detected per colonoscopy.[4] Since that time, 5 additional prospective, randomized trials have been published that have aimed to examine the efficacy of applying CADe to colonoscopy using deep learning methods. In a recent meta-analysis of 6 randomized clinical trials using deep convolutional neural network (CNN)-based CADe systems, Mohan and colleagues[11] found a significantly higher pooled ADR of 32.8% (95% CI, 24.2–42.7) using CADe compared with 21.1% (95% CI, 14.5–29.7; risk ratio [RR] = 1.5; 95% CI, 1.3 to 1.72; $P<.0001$) using standard colonoscopy. The investigators found per-patient adenoma detection parameters were also better using CADe colonoscopy and that withdrawal time increased with a mean difference of 0.38 minutes (95% CI, 0.05–0.72; $P=.02$). Barua and colleagues[12] and Hassan and colleagues[13] found similar results in recent meta-analyses of 5 prospective CADe trials.

Computer-Aided Detection in the Endoscopy Suite: Technical and Practical Considerations

As the evidence for CADe during colonoscopy mounts, it will become increasingly important for endoscopists to familiarize themselves with the technology. Important considerations include monitor setup, processor configuration, and intraprocedural use.[14]

Regarding monitor setup, the CADe output can be deployed in either a single- or a dual-monitor configuration. In the single-monitor configuration, the CADe output is integrated into the output of the primary endoscopy monitor (**Fig. 1**). In the dual-monitor configuration, a second monitor is deployed adjacent to the primary endoscopy monitor. This monitor displays the standard colonoscopy video output in addition to the CADe output. Although the dual-monitor setup was used in many of the first prospective clinical trials,[4,15] a single-monitor configuration may be preferred in the clinical setting so that the endoscopist can focus on a single screen. In order for this to be practical and feasible, however, the screen latency, which can be introduced by certain CADe systems (ie, the few milliseconds required for a computer to process video and identify polyp location), must be below a common detectable threshold.[15] If latency is greater, a dual-screen setup may be preferred to minimize distraction during endoscopy. A dual-screen configuration, in turn, may negatively affect physician gaze patterns and take attention away from the primary monitor.[16] Regarding processor setup, most existing CADe systems use an additional processor that either sits within a mobile cart adjacent to the primary colonoscopy equipment tower or that is small enough to add to the primary setup. In the future, we expect to see remote, cloud-based systems as well as systems that are directly incorporated into the endoscopy processor.

Once the endoscopist has started a procedure using CADe during colonoscopy, they should consider several key concepts. Conventional CADe output is typically in the form of a hollow, bounded box that serves as a visual alarm (**Fig. 2**), although other visual outputs can be used, and some CADe systems also use an optional audio alarm.[17] In order to ensure that a CADe system is performing optimally, the endoscopist must use good mucosal inspection techniques, including adequate insufflation of the colonic lumen during withdrawal, adequate suction to clear away fluid and debris, use of simethicone to limit foam, and limiting inadvertent "suction polyps."[10,14] Underinflation or utilization of CADe before adequate clearance of debris will lead to unnecessary and distracting false positives (**Fig. 3**). In addition, the endoscopist will likely prefer to use the primary monitor output during insertion and during biopsy,

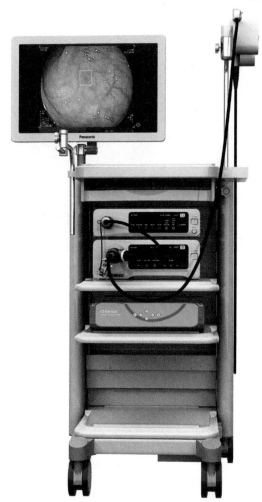

Fig. 1. A CADe system, GI-Genius (Medtronic) with a single-monitor configuration. *Courtesy of* Medtronic, Minneapolis, MN.

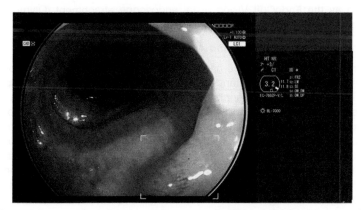

Fig. 2. Output from a representative CADe system (Fujifilm Corp). In this case, the visual alarm is represented by a hollow, bounded box. *Courtesy of* Fujifilm Corp, Tokyo, JP.

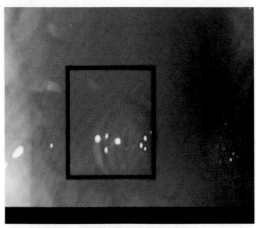

Fig. 3. A false positive. In this case, the CADe system has deployed a visual alarm over a bubble. False positives can be minimized by using good-practice mucosal inspection techniques, such as adequate insufflation, use of suction, use of washing, and use of simethicone when appropriate.

polypectomy, and other endoscopic interventions to avoid potential distraction from stray indicator boxes. For two-screen configurations, the endoscopist may choose to have the second monitor turned away from the visual field until withdrawal begins, and for single-monitor configurations, the endoscopist may choose to toggle CADe "off" during insertion and endoscopic intervention and "on" during most of withdrawal if a toggle feature is available for a given CADe system.[10] It is important to note that even with optimal mucosal inspection, false positives may still occasionally be encountered. These false positives usually represent artifacts within the bowel wall, flecks of stool, or bubbles.[15,18] In addition, the frequency of false positives varies significantly in the literature depending on the clinical definition used.[19] CADe during colonoscopy is a useful tool for highlighting lesions that appear in the visual field but might otherwise go undetected by the human operator. It does not address lesions that remain outside of the visual field, such as polyps behind a mucosal fold. In the future, CADe may be paired with devices that enhance the ability to visualize the mucosa, such as the EndoCuff Vision distal endoscope attachment (Olympus Corp, Tokyo, Japan).[14,20]

Computer-Aided Detection: Emerging Applications

In addition to colonoscopy, CADe has been used for a variety of other applications within gastroenterology. For instance, CADe has been applied to upper endoscopy for the detection of Barrett's esophagus (BE) and esophageal malignancy. BE can often be subtle on white-light upper endoscopy, and dysplasia or early esophageal adenocarcinoma can also go undetected by the untrained eye. This leads to a substantial subset of BE and esophageal cancers that go missed by the endoscopist every year.[21] Advanced endoscopic imaging modalities, such as endomicroscopy, narrow band imaging, and volumetric laser endomicroscopy, have led to improvements in lesion recognition by human endoscopists, but these techniques are often used in specialized settings and are subject to significant interoperator variability.[22,23] Deep learning-based CADe systems trained either on white light or on specialized images are a potential solution to both of these issues. Like other CADe technologies, early studies for the use of CADe in upper GI malignancies consisted of publishing training, validation, and test data on still images and/or video data for a variety of pre-cancerous and cancerous lesions, such as esophageal squamous cell carcinoma, Barrett's esophagus-related neoplasia (BERN), gastric atrophy, gastric intestinal metaplasia, and gastric adenocarcinoma (GCA).[24] In one of the earliest prospective, clinical studies examining CADe for upper GI lesions, Luo and colleagues[24] trained and tested a deep learning CNN on 1,036,496 endoscopy images from 84,424 individuals from 6 hospitals in China. More recently, de Groof and colleagues[25] published development and validation data for a deep learning algorithm built on a hybrid ResNet-UNet CNN as well as pilot study data using this CADe system prospectively during white-light upper endoscopy.[26] The CADe system classified still images as containing neoplasm or nondysplastic BE with an accuracy of 89%, sensitivity of 90%, and specificity of 88%.[25] In the follow-up prospective pilot study, the CADe system detected neoplasia in 9 of 10 patients and produced a false positive in 1 of 10 patients.[26] In a recent meta-analysis of 19 studies using CADe for upper GI neoplasia, including those by Luo and colleagues, and de Groof and colleagues, Arribas and colleagues[23] found a pooled sensitivity of 90% (CI, 85% to 94%), specificity of 89% (CI, 85% to 92%), positive predictive value of 87% (CI, 83% to 91%), and negative predictive value (NPV) of 91% (CI, 87% to 94%), for the detection of esophageal squamous cell carcinoma, BERN, and GCA. It is important to note, however, that the investigators found that current study quality was low with a high risk of selection bias. In a similar meta-analysis, Lui and colleagues found similarly high-performance characteristics for the detection of stomach neoplasia, BERN, squamous cell carcinoma, and *Helicobacter pylori* in early studies.[27] In the near future, we will likely see the publication of high-quality, multicenter, randomized clinical trials applying CADe to upper GI malignancy.

CADe has also successfully been applied to lesion detection during capsule endoscopy (CE).[28] Thus far, CADe algorithms have been developed for the detection of protruding lesions, such as polyps in the small bowel,[29] angioectasias,[30] inflammation, ulcers, polyps, parasites,[31,32] and celiac-related small bowel enteropathy.[33] Interestingly, AI has also successfully been applied for capsule location in differentiating between stomach, small bowel, and colon with 96% accuracy.[34,35] The study of AI applied to CE is in its infancy, and current studies are based on training and validation on still images. We will soon likely see the prospective application of such systems in clinical and commercial contexts, and the expectation is that AI may substantially improve the efficiency of the otherwise laborious task of capsule review by physicians.

COMPUTER-AIDED DIAGNOSIS
History and Evidence: Computer-Aided Diagnosis

In addition to CADe, CADx is the second area of intense investigation within the subfield of AI as applied to gastroenterology. CADx or *optical biopsy* is the use of computational analysis to predict histology without the need for conventional tissue biopsy.[36] The field of optical biopsy is several decades old, but the recent utilization of deep learning techniques has led to important recent developments in this space. The European Society of Gastrointestinal Endoscopy currently recommends the use of virtual and dye-based chromoendoscopy as an alternative to biopsy or resection of diminutive polyps in the rectosigmoid colon,[35,37] and endocytoscopy, an advanced imaging modality that uses in situ magnification of up to 520 times of images of the surface epithelium during endoscopy, has also been used to predict polyp histology.[38] Many of these techniques have proven effective when used by experts in specialized academic centers, but performance characteristics degrade when they are not used by experts.[38] AI and deep learning systems have the potential to decrease interoperator variability and allow these technologies to reach important diagnostic thresholds when used by endoscopists of varying skill levels.[39–41] CADx systems for automatic characterization of polyp histology during colonoscopy have been developed for use with magnifying Narrow Band Imaging (NBI), endocytoscopy, laser autofluorescence, and white-light images, but this field is still in its infancy. Currently, there are 6 prospective studies examining CADx during colonoscopy. only one of these prospective studies involves more than 100 patients, and no randomized, clinical trials yet exist.[36,41] Four of these studies used CADx systems developed on images from autofluorescence endoscopy; one used a CADx system developed on output from magnifying NBI, and one study used a system built on images from endocytoscopy. An example of a CADx system developed on endocytoscopy images can be seen in **Fig. 4**. The largest study, published by Mori and colleagues[41] in 2019, was a prospective, single-arm, open-label study that involved the use of a CADx algorithm previously developed using endocytoscopy images from 5 endoscopy centers in Japan that predicted polyp histology ("neoplastic" or "nonneoplastic") in NBI and stained modes using an endocytoscopy system capable of 520× magnification. Polyp prediction by the CADx algorithm was compared with pathology analysis of resected polyps. Seven hundred ninety-one consecutive patients undergoing colonoscopy by 23 endoscopists at a single endoscopy center in Japan were involved. The primary end point was whether CADx with the stained mode produced a NPV of 90% or greater for identifying diminutive rectosigmoid adenomas. The investigators found an NPV of 93.7% to 96.5% (95% CI, 88.3% to 97.1%; CI, 92.1% to 98.9%) depending on assumptions made about polyps lacking either a CADx or a histopathologic diagnosis. Although this study was not a randomized clinical trial, it was revolutionary in that it was the largest trial to involve a CADx system prospectively, and the results reached the diagnostic threshold to support the "diagnose and leave" strategy laid out by the American Society for Gastrointestinal Endoscopy (ASGE) Preservation and Incorporation of Valuable Endoscopic Innovations-2 initiative. This posits that a technology should provide a diagnostic threshold of ≥90% NPV for adenomatous polyp histology for that technology to support diagnosis of a rectosigmoid polyp as nonadenomatous/

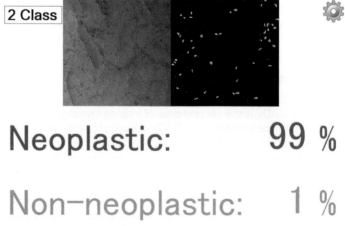

Fig. 4. A CADx system for use during colonoscopy. This system was trained on endocytoscopy images. Output predicts nonneoplastic versus neoplastic histology based on surface features. *Courtesy of* Yuichi Mori MD, PhD, Oslo, NO.

nonmalignant and leave it in place without removal.[42] CADx has also been used to further characterize BE as nondysplastic versus dysplastic, as can be seen in **Fig. 5**.

Novel applications of CADx in gastroenterology also include endoscopic and radiographic imaging analysis. One of the earliest applications of AI in clinical medicine involved the use of CADx in histopathology and imaging.[43,44] In gastroenterology, applications in pathology have included the use of deep learning to classify upper GI biopsies as adenocarcinoma, adenoma, and nonneoplastic[45]; duodenal biopsies as celiac disease versus environmental enteropathy versus normal[46]; and pancreatic cyst fluid as coming from malignant versus benign pancreatic cysts.[47] In imaging, deep learning has been used for the automatic segment of CT enterography images in Crohn disease in order to predict stricturing versus nonstricturing disease,[48] the differentiation of autoimmune pancreatitis from pancreatic cancer in endoscopic ultrasound (EUS), and the characterization of focal lesions of the liver on EUS.[49] CADx has also been used to automate endoscopic severity scores in ulcerative colitis.[50]

FUTURE DIRECTIONS
Combined Modalities

Preliminary data have also been published on "full-workflow" systems combining complex detection and classification algorithms. Work from Mori and colleagues[51] seeks to combine CADe and CADx using endocytoscopy. In 2019, Guizard and colleagues[52] published preliminary data on a combined system that detected and tracked polyps during colonoscopy video and had the ability to perform optical biopsy on multiple polyps that appeared in the same frame. The system was also able to apply unique labels to each polyp, which could be revisited later in the procedure. Systems such as these, which combine multiple AI-based functions into 1 user-friendly output, are likely the way forward in the future for AI in GI endoscopy. Additional publications examining the efficacy, feasibility, effectiveness, and cost of such systems in the future are eagerly awaited.

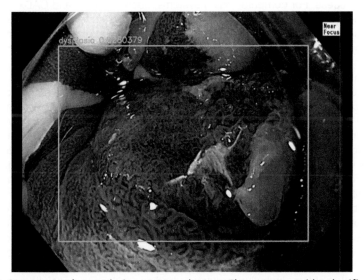

Fig. 5. A CADx system for use during upper endoscopy. The system provides classification of dysplastic versus nondysplastic and outputs localization boxes around regions classified as dysplasia. *Courtesy of* DocBot, Redwood City, CA.

Operations, Decision Support, and Quality Improvement

AI also has the potential to optimize day-to-day workflow and decision making in clinical medicine and in endoscopy. Through integration with the electronic medical record (EMR), AI is uniquely positioned to automate routine tasks, such as the pre-review of laboratory data and imaging results.[53] In addition, natural language processing prototypes exist that have the potential to compile health records and optimize clinical note taking.[53] Systems that use ambient clinical intelligence, AI used to monitor and react to auditory or visual stimuli, will also likely be used to document clinical encounters and augment postendoscopy documentation without explicit dictation.[54]

AI has been applied to the streamlining of nearly every step of endoscopy. There are nascent efforts to use AI to automatically document and generate endoscopy reports, and there are already publications using AI to recognize and label endoscopy landmarks, measure withdrawal time, record bowel preparation quality, and recognize endoscopic intervention.[54,55] Deep learning has also been successfully applied to quality assurance in endoscopy to minimize blind spots in upper endoscopy and colonoscopy.[56,57] AI/ML has been used to generate prediction models for a variety of clinical problems encountered in gastroenterology from variables associated with an inflammatory bowel disease flare,[58] to determining risk in patients presenting with upper GI bleed,[59] to predicting the presence of lymph node metastasis in T1 colorectal cancers.[60] Future iterations of the EMR will likely integrate heterogenous sources of data from medical literature, public databases, claims reports, and clinical encounters with validated prediction models to help drive both research and clinical care.

IMPLEMENTATION, COMMERCIALIZATION, REGULATION, AND POTENTIAL PITFALLS
Implementation and Commercialization

As data about the efficacy and potential usefulness of various AI-based technologies continue to accumulate, new questions about cost-effectiveness and implementation will continue to be raised. Going from algorithm development to commercialization is a complex process. For computer vision systems, such as CADe and CADx technologies, going from the computer bench to the endoscopy suite will involve algorithm development, clinical translation, head-to-head comparison of seemingly similar systems, production-grade integration into the endoscope, demonstration of improved outcomes (and potentially reduced costs), ultimate commercialization, and ongoing regulation.[61]

Before clinical implementation, individual computer vision systems should ideally be tested prospectively in large, randomized clinical trials. Because each system may be improved iteratively through use and because several similar algorithms may emerge by different groups, it will become increasingly important for there to be a means of directly comparing computer vision systems to previous versions and to different algorithms with similar applications. Existing systems may be tested "head-to-head" in multiarm, randomized trials, although this may not be practical or feasible as more similar systems are developed. An alternative is to test existing systems on standardized benchmark data sets: large, heterogenous, curated data sets with broad representation in terms of lesion type and presentation.[5,62] Thus far, several such candidate databases exist.[62,63] It is likely that national and international endoscopy societies will play a major role in the future in curating these databases and certifying new technologies.

Many stakeholders, including regulatory bodies, endoscopy societies, insurance providers, practice managers, and individual physicians, will also need to think critically about the cost-effectiveness of any AI technology before considering its integration into the endoscopy suite. In a recent add-on analysis to Mori and colleagues' prospective CADx endocytoscopy study,[41] Mori and colleagues found that using CADx to support a diagnose and disregard strategy was favorable in a detailed cost-benefit analysis.[64] The investigators compared the use of CADx during colonoscopy to support a diagnose and leave strategy (assuming that all diminutive rectosigmoid polyps that were predicted as nonneoplastic by the AI system were left in situ) with standard colonoscopy without the use of AI, using a resect-all-polyps strategy. The investigators did not include the cost of anesthesia or sedation in their analysis. They estimated that the initial purchase fee of the CADx technology for an endoscopy unit in Japan was US$46,119; the implementation fee was US$1820, and the annual maintenance fee was US$1092 for a total of US$49,031. Assuming that the CADx system was used on 1000 cases annually for 5 consecutive years, the per-colonoscopy cost was estimated to be US$10. Mori and colleagues[64] found that in Japan the cost of colonoscopy using CADx to support a diagnose and leave strategy was US$119 lower than the resect all polyps strategy using Japanese reimbursement rates, US$52 lower in the United Kingdom, US$34 lower in Norway, and US$125 lower in the United States based on Medicare reimbursement rates. The expected gross annual reimbursement savings for colonoscopy was estimated to be US$85,244,220.[64] The investigators concluded that implementation of AI-assisted optical biopsy was cost-effective, and clinical implementation should be encouraged, as should reimbursement support from public and private insurance bodies. In the United States, there are additional considerations. For instance, routine use of CADx could reduce downstream revenue to pathology laboratories, which is an important revenue source for some private gastroenterology practices, ambulatory centers, and hospitals.

Regulation and Potential Pitfalls

As CADe and CADx technologies continue to grow and evolve, there is a parallel need for regulatory pathways to evolve and directly address the new, unique challenges that come with applying AI/ML to clinical care.[65] In the United States, algorithms will likely be regulated as "software as a medical device" categorized from low to high risk (4 risk categories total) based on framework established by the International Medical Device Regulators Forum. Under the current FDA framework, CADe and CADx tools will likely be classified as class II devices because they are of moderate risk and complex in design but do not sustain life and are not implantable.[65] It is likely that a framework will first evolve for "locked" algorithms, which have fixed performance characteristics and that additional complexity will be added with technology that is designed to learn and evolve autonomously.[65] Between 2020 and 2021, several CADe and CADx systems gained regulatory approval in Japan and Europe, including GI-Genius (Medtronic, Minneapolis, MN, USA), CAD-EYE (Fujifilm Corp, Tokyo, Japan), DISCOVERY (Pentax Corp, Tokyo, Japan), Endo-BRAIN-Plus (Olympus), EndoBRAIN-EYE (Olympus), and ENDO-AID (Olympus). In April 2021, the FDA announced the first U.S. regulatory approval for a CADe polyp detection system (GI-Genius), and soon U.S. gastroenterologists will likely have multiple CADe systems to choose from. Before implementation, a variety of potential barriers and ethical challenges must also be addressed, including lack of AI model interpretability, overstatement of AI benefits owing to inappropriate comparisons between a given algorithm to a clinical baseline, low uptake despite proven benefit, ambiguity surrounding liability in cases of harm, and potential exacerbation of inequities in gender, sex, and ethnicity because of inadvertent biased algorithm development.[66]

SUMMARY

In conclusion, AI promises to optimize workflow and change the way that we practice in the endoscopy suite and in the clinic in myriad ways. CADe will likely be incorporated into endoscopy suites across the world for use during colonoscopy as a second set of eyes within the next 1 to 2 years, and both CADe and CADx hold the promise of decreasing interoperator variability with standard and specialized technologies and improving clinical care. As evidence for these technologies continues to accumulate, it will become increasingly important for gastroenterologists to familiarize themselves with the evidence, the terminology, and the benefits and limitations of AI, ML, and deep learning.

CLINICS CARE POINTS

- The field of gastroenterology has applied artificial intelligence to a vast array of clinical problems, and some of the earliest prospective trials examining artificial intelligence in medicine have been in computer vision applied to endoscopy.
- Evidence is mounting for 2 broad areas of application in regards to artificial intelligence as applied to gastroenterology: computer-aided detection and computer-aided diagnosis.
- For computer-aided detection, multiple recent prospective trials have shown a substantial increase in adenoma detection rate when a computer-aided detection system is used in comparison to white-light colonoscopy alone.
- When using computer-aided detection, the endoscopist needs to consider single- versus dual-monitor configurations. A single-screen setup may be preferred in the clinical setting.
- In order to ensure that a computer-aided detection system is performing optimally, the endoscopist must use good mucosal inspection techniques, including adequate insufflation of the colonic lumen during withdrawal, adequate suction, use of simethicone to limit foam, and limiting inadvertent "suction polyps."
- It is important to note that even with optimal mucosal inspection, false positives may still occasionally be encountered. These usually represent artifacts within the bowel wall, flecks of stool, or bubbles.
- Computer-aided detection has also been studied in the setting of upper endoscopy for the detection of various malignant and premalignant conditions. Computer-aided detection has the potential to decrease interobserver variability, especially on systems trained using advanced imaging modalities, such as endocytoscopy, narrow band imaging, and volumetric laser endomicroscopy, which are often used in specialized settings.
- Evidence is mounting for the use of computer-aided diagnosis as well, and recent prospective work suggests that a computer-aided diagnosis system based on endocytoscopy may support a "diagnose and leave" strategy for diminutive polyps in the rectosigmoid colon.
- "Full-workflow" systems combining complex detection and classification algorithms will likely be the way forward in the future.
- Artificial intelligence also has the potential to optimize day-to-day workflow and decision making in clinical medicine and in endoscopy.

DISCLOSURE

Tyler Berzin has served as a consultant for Wision AI, Fujifilm, and Medtronic. The remaining author has no conflicts of interest to disclose.

REFERENCES

1. Phene S, Dunn RC, Hammel N, et al. Deep learning and glaucoma specialists: the relative importance of optic disc features to predict glaucoma referral in fundus photographs. Ophthalmology 2019;126(12):1627–39.
2. Shen L, Margolies LR, Rothstein JH, et al. Deep learning to improve breast cancer detection on screening mammography. Sci Rep 2019;9(1):12495.
3. Han SS, Kim MS, Lim W, et al. Classification of the clinical images for benign and malignant cutaneous tumors using a deep learning algorithm. J Invest Dermatol 2018;138(7):1529–38.
4. Wang P, Berzin TM, Glissen Brown JR, et al. Real-time automatic detection system increases colonoscopic polyp and adenoma detection rates: a prospective randomised controlled study. Gut 2019;68(10):1813–9.
5. van der Sommen F, de Groof J, Struyvenberg M, et al. Machine learning in GI endoscopy: practical guidance in how to interpret a novel field. Gut 2020; 69(11):2035–45.
6. Chartrand G, Cheng PM, Vorontsov E, et al. Deep learning: a primer for radiologists. Radiographics 2017;37(7):2113–31.
7. Iakovidis DK, Maroulis DE, Karkanis SA. An intelligent system for automatic detection of gastrointestinal adenomas in video endoscopy. Comput Biol Med 2006;36(10):1084–103.
8. Karkanis S, Galousi K, Maroulis D. Classification of endoscopic images based on texture spectrum. ACAI99, Workshop on Machine Learning in Medical Applications 2000.
9. Wang Y, Tavanapong W, Wong J, et al. Polyp-Alert: near real-time feedback during colonoscopy. Comput Methods Programs Biomed 2015;120(3):164–79.
10. Bilal M, Glissen Brown JR, Berzin TM. Using computer-aided polyp detection during colonoscopy. Am J Gastroenterol 2020;115(7):963–6.
11. Mohan BP, Facciorusso A, Khan SR, et al. Real-time computer aided colonoscopy versus standard colonoscopy for improving adenoma detection rate: a meta-analysis of randomized-controlled trials. EClinicalMedicine 2020;29.
12. Hassan C, Spadaccini M, Iannone A, et al. Artificial intelligence for polyp detection during colonoscopy: a systematic review and meta-analysis. Endoscopy 2021;53(3):277–84.
13. Hassan C, Spadaccini M, Iannone A, et al. Performance of artificial intelligence in colonoscopy for adenoma and polyp detection: a systematic review and meta-analysis. Gastrointest Endosc 2021;93(1):77-85.e6.
14. Glissen Brown JR, Bilal M, Wang P, et al. Introducing computer-aided detection to the endoscopy suite. VideoGIE 2020;5(4):135–7.
15. Wang P, Liu X, Berzin TM, et al. Effect of a deep-learning computer-aided detection system on adenoma detection during colonoscopy (CADe-DB trial): a double-blind randomised study. Lancet Gastroenterol Hepatol 2020;5(4):343–51.
16. Lami M, Singh H, Dilley JH, et al. Gaze patterns hold key to unlocking successful search strategies and increasing polyp detection rate in colonoscopy. Endoscopy 2018;50(7):701–7.
17. Wang P, Xiao X, Glissen Brown JR, et al. Development and validation of a deep-learning algorithm for the detection of polyps during colonoscopy. Nat Biomed Eng 2018;2(10):741–8.
18. Hassan C, Badalamenti M, Maselli R, et al. Computer-aided detection-assisted colonoscopy: classification and relevance of false positives. Gastrointest Endosc 2020;92(4):900-4.e4.

19. Holzwanger EA, Bilal M, Glissen Brown JR, et al. Benchmarking false positive definitions for computer aided polyp detection in colonoscopy. Endoscopy 2020.

20. Ngu WS, Bevan R, Tsiamoulos ZP, et al. Improved adenoma detection with Endocuff Vision: the ADENOMA randomised controlled trial. Gut 2019;68(2):280–8.

21. Menon S, Trudgill N. How commonly is upper gastrointestinal cancer missed at endoscopy? A meta-analysis. Endosc Int Open 2014;2(2):E46–50.

22. Kikuste I, Marques-Pereira R, Monteiro-Soares M, et al. Systematic review of the diagnosis of gastric premalignant conditions and neoplasia with high-resolution endoscopic technologies. Scand J Gastroenterol 2013;48(10):1108–17.

23. Arribas J, Antonelli G, Frazzoni L, et al. Standalone performance of artificial intelligence for upper GI neoplasia: a meta-analysis. Gut 2020.

24. Luo H, Xu G, Li C, et al. Real-time artificial intelligence for detection of upper gastrointestinal cancer by endoscopy: a multicentre, case-control, diagnostic study. Lancet Oncol 2019;20(12):1645–54.

25. de Groof AJ, Struyvenberg MR, van der Putten J, et al. Deep-learning system detects neoplasia in patients with Barrett's esophagus with higher accuracy than endoscopists in a multistep training and validation study with benchmarking. Gastroenterology 2020;158(4):915–29.e914.

26. de Groof AJ, Struyvenberg MR, Fockens KN, et al. Deep learning algorithm detection of Barrett's neoplasia with high accuracy during live endoscopic procedures: a pilot study (with video). Gastrointest Endosc 2020;91(6):1242–50.

27. Lui TKL, Tsui VWM, Leung WK. Accuracy of artificial intelligence-assisted detection of upper GI lesions: a systematic review and meta-analysis. *Gastrointest Endosc* 2020;92(4):821–830.e9.

28. Glissen Brown JR, Berzin TM. Deploying artificial intelligence to find the needle in the haystack: deep learning for video capsule endoscopy. Gastrointest Endosc 2020;92(1):152–3.

29. Saito H, Aoki T, Aoyama K, et al. Automatic detection and classification of protruding lesions in wireless capsule endoscopy images based on a deep convolutional neural network. Gastrointest Endosc 2020;92(1):144–51.e141.

30. Leenhardt R, Vasseur P, Li C, et al. A neural network algorithm for detection of GI angiectasia during small-bowel capsule endoscopy. Gastrointest Endosc 2019; 89(1):189–94.

31. Ding Z, Shi H, Zhang H, et al. Gastroenterologist-level identification of small-bowel diseases and normal variants by capsule endoscopy using a deep-learning model. Gastroenterology 2019;157(4):1044–54.e1045.

32. He J, Wu X, Jiang Y, et al. Hookworm detection in wireless capsule endoscopy images with deep learning. IEEE Trans Image Process 2018;27(5):2379–92.

33. Zhou W, Yang M, Wang X, et al. Scalable feature matching by dual cascaded scalar quantization for image retrieval. IEEE Trans Pattern Anal Mach Intell 2016;38(1):159–71.

34. Zou Y, Li L, Wang Y, et al. Classifying digestive organs in wireless capsule endoscopy images based on deep convolutional neural network. Paper presented at: 2015 IEEE International Conference on Digital Signal Processing (DSP); 21-24 July 2015 2015.

35. Chahal D, Byrne MF. A primer on artificial intelligence and its application to endoscopy. Gastrointest Endosc 2020;92(4):813–20.e814.

36. Alagappan M, Brown JRG, Mori Y, et al. Artificial intelligence in gastrointestinal endoscopy: the future is almost here. World J Gastrointest Endosc 2018; 10(10):239–49.

37. Bisschops R, East JE, Hassan C, et al. Advanced imaging for detection and differentiation of colorectal neoplasia: European Society of Gastrointestinal Endoscopy (ESGE) Guideline - update 2019. Endoscopy 2019;51(12):1155–79.
38. Inoue H, Kudo SE, Shiokawa A. Technology insight: laser-scanning confocal microscopy and endocytoscopy for cellular observation of the gastrointestinal tract. Nat Clin Pract Gastroenterol Hepatol 2005;2(1):31–7.
39. Chen P-J, Lin M-C, Lai M-J, et al. Accurate classification of diminutive colorectal polyps using computer-aided analysis. Gastroenterology 2018;154(3):568–75.
40. Byrne MF, Chapados N, Soudan F, et al. Real-time differentiation of adenomatous and hyperplastic diminutive colorectal polyps during analysis of unaltered videos of standard colonoscopy using a deep learning model. Gut 2019;68(1):94.
41. Mori Y, Kudo SE, Misawa M, et al. Real-time use of artificial intelligence in identification of diminutive polyps during colonoscopy: a prospective study. Ann Intern Med 2018;169(6):357–66.
42. Committee AT, Abu Dayyeh BK, Thosani N, et al. ASGE Technology Committee systematic review and meta-analysis assessing the ASGE PIVI thresholds for adopting real-time endoscopic assessment of the histology of diminutive colorectal polyps. Gastrointest Endosc 2015;81(3):502.e501–16.
43. Elter M, Horsch A. CADx of mammographic masses and clustered microcalcifications: a review. Med Phys 2009;36(6):2052–68.
44. Bengtsson E, Danielsen H, Treanor D, et al. Computer-aided diagnostics in digital pathology. Cytometry A 2017;91(6):551–4.
45. Iizuka O, Kanavati F, Kato K, et al. Deep learning models for histopathological classification of gastric and colonic epithelial tumours. Sci Rep 2020;10(1):1504.
46. Syed S, Al-Boni M, Khan MN, et al. Assessment of machine learning detection of environmental enteropathy and celiac disease in children. JAMA Netw Open 2019;2(6):e195822.
47. Kurita Y, Kuwahara T, Hara K, et al. Diagnostic ability of artificial intelligence using deep learning analysis of cyst fluid in differentiating malignant from benign pancreatic cystic lesions. Sci Rep 2019;9(1):6893.
48. Stidham RW, Enchakalody B, Waljee AK, et al. Assessing small bowel stricturing and morphology in Crohn's disease using semi-automated image analysis. Inflamm Bowel Dis 2020;26(5):734–42.
49. Marya NB, Powers PD, Fujii-Lau L, et al. Application of artificial intelligence using a novel EUS-based convolutional neural network model to identify and distinguish benign and malignant hepatic masses. Gastrointest Endosc 2021;93(5): 1121–1130.e1.
50. Takenaka K, Ohtsuka K, Fujii T, et al. Development and validation of a deep neural network for accurate evaluation of endoscopic images from patients with ulcerative colitis. Gastroenterology 2020;158(8):2150–7.
51. Mori Y, Kudo S-e, Misawa M, et al. Simultaneous detection and characterization of diminutive polyps with the use of artificial intelligence during colonoscopy. VideoGIE 2019;4(1):7–10.
52. Guizard N, Ghalehjegh SH, Henkel M, et al. 256 – Artificial intelligence for real-time multiple polyp detection with identification, tracking, and optical biopsy during colonoscopy. Gastroenterology 2019;156(6). S-48-S-49.
53. Reddy S, Fox J, Purohit MP. Artificial intelligence-enabled healthcare delivery. J R Soc Med 2019;112(1):22–8.
54. Berzin TM, Parasa S, Wallace MB, Gross SA, Repici A, Sharma P. Position statement on priorities for artificial intelligence in GI endoscopy: a report by the ASGE Task Force. Gastrointest Endosc 2020;92(4):951–9.

55. Zhou J, Wu L, Wan X, et al. A novel artificial intelligence system for the assessment of bowel preparation (with video). Gastrointest Endosc 2020;91(2): 428–35.e422.

56. Thakkar S, Carleton NM, Rao B, et al. Use of artificial intelligence-based analytics from live colonoscopies to optimize the quality of the colonoscopy examination in real time: proof of concept. Gastroenterology 2020;158(5):1219–21.e1212.

57. Wu L, Zhang J, Zhou W, et al. Randomised controlled trial of WISENSE, a real-time quality improving system for monitoring blind spots during esophagogastroduodenoscopy. Gut 2019;68(12):2161–9.

58. Waljee AK, Lipson R, Wiitala WL, et al. Predicting hospitalization and outpatient corticosteroid use in inflammatory bowel disease patients using machine learning. Inflamm Bowel Dis 2017;24(1):45–53.

59. Shung DL, Au B, Taylor RA, et al. Validation of a machine learning model that outperforms clinical risk scoring systems for upper gastrointestinal bleeding. Gastroenterology 2020;158(1):160–7.

60. Kudo S-E, Ichimasa K, Villard B, et al. Artificial intelligence system to determine risk of T1 colorectal cancer metastasis to lymph node. Gastroenterology 2021; 160(4):1075–84.e2.

61. Parasa S, Wallace M, Bagci U, et al. Proceedings from the first global artificial intelligence in gastroenterology and endoscopy summit. Gastrointest Endosc 2020;92(4):938–45.e1.

62. Misawa M, Kudo S-E, Mori Y, et al. Development of a computer-aided detection system for colonoscopy and a publicly accessible large colonoscopy video database (With video). *Gastrointest Endosc* 2021;93(4):960–967.e3.

63. Borgli H, Thambawita V, Smedsrud PH, et al. HyperKvasir, a comprehensive multi-class image and video dataset for gastrointestinal endoscopy. Scientific Data 2020;7(1):283.

64. Mori Y, Kudo SE, East JE, et al. Cost savings in colonoscopy with artificial intelligence-aided polyp diagnosis: an add-on analysis of a clinical trial (with video). Gastrointest Endosc 2020;92(4):905–11.e1.

65. Walradt T, Glissen Brown JR, Alagappan M, et al. Regulatory considerations for artificial intelligence technologies in GI endoscopy. Gastrointest Endosc 2020; 92(4):801–6.

66. Vollmer S, Mateen BA, Bohner G, et al. Machine learning and artificial intelligence research for patient benefit: 20 critical questions on transparency, replicability, ethics, and effectiveness. BMJ 2020;368:l6927.

Role of Anesthesia in Endoscopic Operations

Yoon-Jeong Cho, MD

KEYWORDS

- Anesthesia for endoscopy • Preanesthetic assessment • ASA status
- Conscious sedation • Monitored anesthesia care • Non–operating room anesthesia

KEY POINTS

- Although most endoscopic operations can be safely performed under conscious sedation, there are indications for general anesthesia with endotracheal intubation.
- A thorough preanesthetic assessment in the context of specific patient and procedure should direct the appropriate depth of sedation or type of anesthesia.
- Whether a patient should require anesthesia care should be assessed in advance and incorporated into scheduling to improve efficiency in endoscopy suites.
- A team-based approach and good communication between the proceduralist and anesthesia care team improve efficiency and quality of patient care.

INTRODUCTION

Gastrointestinal (GI) endoscopic operations have seen significant advancements and increase in technical complexity[1,2] along with increasing comorbidities and medical complexity of patient population[3] over the past decade. Several of these operations are frequently performed in outpatient settings with nonoperating room anesthesia.[3–5] Utilization of anesthesia providers has become increasingly common in both smaller, private practice settings to university hospitals and tertiary centers over the years.[6,7] Some of the advanced endoscopic procedures are associated with longer procedural times and require patient cooperation, especially if no or only minimal sedation is used. They can result in patient discomfort and pain from various reasons from the nature of the procedure itself, such as insufflation, triggering of the gag reflex by the introduction of the endoscope, the disease process itself, or from patient positioning. Patients who are tolerant to anxiolytics and sedatives may also experience significant discomfort when a procedure is attempted with minimal sedation/anxiolysis. This in turn can result in difficulty in completing the procedure or further prolong the procedural time, potentially leading to a suboptimal procedure and/or decrease in patient satisfaction.

Department of General Anesthesiology, Cleveland Clinic, 9500 Euclid Avenue, Cleveland, OH 44195, USA
E-mail address: choy@ccf.org

Gastrointest Endoscopy Clin N Am 31 (2021) 759–772
https://doi.org/10.1016/j.giec.2021.05.011
1052-5157/21/© 2021 Elsevier Inc. All rights reserved.
giendo.theclinics.com

The availability and utilization of anesthesia providers can facilitate procedural needs and may also increase patient satisfaction.[8–10] In addition, anesthesiologists can focus on management of the airway and hemodynamics for patients with significant comorbidities and complicated medical history (**Table 1**), allowing the endoscopists to focus on the procedural aspects.

In this section, the author discuss the preanesthetic/preprocedural evaluation with a focus on factors that should be considered in choosing the level of sedation or type of anesthesia, patient monitoring, and necessary equipment, followed by an overview of postanesthesia care.

PREANESTHETIC/PREPROCEDURAL EVALUATIONS

Preanesthetic evaluations begin with thorough review of the patient's history and physical examination. In addition, special attention is paid to airway assessment and patient's nothing by mouth *nil per os* (NPO) status. In addition to the usual assessments, specific factors that should be considered in anesthetic planning in endoscopic operations include, but are not limited to, the following:

- Procedural factors
  - Type of procedure and indications
  - Expected duration of the procedure
    - Example: patient with known history of multiple colonic polyps scheduled for endoscopic resection
  - Expected difficulties
    - Example: patient with history of multiple abdominal surgeries
  - Positioning of the patient

Table 1
Examples of significant comorbidities that affect anesthetic management and patient outcome of an endoscopic operation

System	Comorbidities
Cardiovascular	• Ischemic heart disease • Congestive heart failure • Presence of devices such as pacemakers, implantable cardiovascular defibrillators, left ventricular assist device, extracorporeal membrane oxygenation • History of significant arrythmia
Respiratory	• Chronic obstructive pulmonary disease (COPD) • Obstructive sleep apnea (OSA) • Severe asthma
Gastrointestinal	• Severe gastroesophageal reflux disease (GERD) • Active gastrointestinal bleeding • Motility disorders, such as achalasia or gastroparesis • Structural abnormalities, such as Zenker's diverticulum • Intestinal obstruction • Liver failure with or without ascites, bleeding esophageal varices
Neurologic	• Cerebrovascular disease

- ■ Example: patient with history of chronic shoulder pain that needs lateral positioning for optimal endoscopic views
  - ○ Possibility of complications in higher risk procedures
- • Patient factors
  - ○ Medical history and comorbidities, as discussed in **Table 1**
- • Urgency or emergency procedure
  - ○ Example: active upper GI bleeding that places patient at a high risk of aspiration with need for intraoperative transfusion and resuscitation

American Society of Anesthesiologists (ASA) Physical Status

American Society of Anesthesiologists physical status (ASA PS, or ASA status) is used to classify a patient's preanesthetic comorbidities (**Table 2**). ASA class system has been in use for more than 60 years and has been revised over time. Although it is not a complete preoperative assessment in itself and may be susceptible to individual provider's subjectivity, its association with postoperative morbidity and mortality has been demonstrated in multiple studies.[11] Enestvedt and colleagues[12] conducted a retrospective cohort analysis of 1.3 million adult patients that underwent endoscopic procedures and found that higher ASA class was associated with increased risk of adverse events, particularly for esophagogastroduodenoscopy (EGD) and colonoscopy. Another retrospective database review conducted by Sharma and colleagues[13] also found a higher incidence of unplanned cardiopulmonary events in patients with higher ASA grade. Interestingly, a survey conducted by Curatolo and colleagues[14] investigated a commonly raised question that nonanesthesia providers often underrate ASA PS. In their study, all surveyed surgical/procedural departments and medicine departments had a 30% to 40% chance of underrating the ASA PS.[14] When ASA PS is being assigned by a nonanesthesia provider, a review of the ASA PS classification and approved examples[15] is helpful for a more accurate prediction of periprocedural morbidity and mortality. Overall, review of a patient's ASA status is a useful tool in preprocedural risk stratification that should be used when determining involvement of anesthesia team.

Nothing by Mouth (NPO) Status

A patient's NPO status is another important component of preoperative evaluation. Induction of general anesthesia results in relaxation of airway muscle tone and blunting of airway reflexes, increasing the risk of pulmonary aspiration. Aspiration can also occur during procedural sedation.[16] ASA has published fasting guidelines to reduce the risk of pulmonary aspiration (**Table 3**[17]).

It should also be noted, however, that these guidelines may need to be modified for patients with conditions that affect gastric emptying or fluid volume (eg, pregnancy, obesity, diabetes, hiatal hernia, GERD, ileus or bowel obstruction, emergency care, or enteral tube feeding),[17] which comprise a good proportion of patients being seen at endoscopy suites. In such situations, a special airway management technique may be pursued (eg, rapid sequence intubation [RSI]) in order to mitigate the risk of aspiration.

Airway Evaluations

Airway management during an upper endoscopic operation poses a unique challenge to the anesthesia or sedation provider because of "shared" upper airway with the proceduralist. Although airway reflexes and spontaneous ventilation are generally unaffected in minimal sedation, deeper level of sedation and general anesthesia

Table 2
American Society of Anesthesiologists physical status classification system

ASA PS Classification	Definition	Adult Examples, Including, but Not Limited to:
ASA I	A normal healthy patient	Healthy, non-smoking, no or minimal alcohol use
ASA II	A patient with mild systemic disease	Mild diseases only without substantive functional limitations. Current smoker, social alcohol drinker, pregnancy, obesity (30 < BMI < 40), well-controlled DM/HTN, mild lung disease
ASA III	A patient with severe systemic disease	Substantive functional limitations; one or more moderate to severe diseases. Poorly controlled DM or HTN, COPD, morbid obesity (BMI $\geq$ 40), active hepatitis, alcohol dependence or abuse, implanted pacemaker, moderate reduction of ejection fraction, ESRD undergoing regularly scheduled dialysis, history (>3 months) of MI, CVA, TIA, or CAD/stents
ASA IV	A patient with severe systemic disease that is a constant threat to life	Recent (<3 months) MI, CVA, TIA, or CAD/stents, ongoing cardiac ischemia or severe valve dysfunction, severe reduction of ejection fraction, shock, sepsis, DIC, ARD, or ESRD not undergoing regularly scheduled dialysis
ASA V	A moribund patient who is not expected to survive without the operation	Ruptured abdominal/thoracic aneurysm, massive trauma, intracranial bleed with mass effect, ischemic bowel in the face of significant cardiac pathology or multiple organ/system dysfunction
ASA VI	A declared brain-dead patient whose organs are being removed for donor purposes	

Abbreviations: ARD, acute respiratory distress; BMI: body mass index; CAD, coronary artery disease; CVA, cerebrovascular accident; DIC, disseminated intravascular coagulation; DM, diabetes mellitus; ESRD, end-stage renal disease; HTN, hypertension; MI, myocardial infarction; PCA, percutaneous coronary angioplasty; TIA, transient ischemic attack.

*Although pregnancy is not a disease, the parturient' s physiologic state is significantly altered from when the woman is not pregnant, hence the assignment of ASA 2 for a woman with uncomplicated pregnancy.

**The addition of "E" denotes Emergency surgery: (An emergency is defined as existing when delay in treatment of the patient would lead to a significant increase in the threat to life or body part).

Excerpted from ASA, ASA Physical Status Classification System (Approved by the ASA House of Delegates on October 15, 2014, and last amended on December 13, 2020) of the American Society of Anesthesiologists. A copy of the full text can be obtained from ASA, 1061 American Lane Schaumburg, IL 60173-4973 or online at www.asahq.org.

Table 3
American Society of Anesthesiologists nothing by mouth guidelines

Ingested Material	Minimum Fasting Period
Clear liquids	2 h
Breast milk	4 h
Infant formula	6 h
Nonhuman milk	6 h
Light meal	6 h
Fried foods, fatty foods, or meat	Additional fasting time (eg, 8 or more hours) may be needed

Excerpted from Practice Guidelines for Preoperative Fasting and the Use of Pharmacologic Agents to Reduce the Risk of Pulmonary Aspiration: Application to Healthy Patients Undergoing Elective Procedures: An Updated Report by the American Society of Anesthesiologists Task Force on Preoperative Fasting and the Use of Pharmacologic Agents to Reduce the Risk of Pulmonary Aspiration. A copy of the full text can be obtained from ASA, 1061 American Lane Schaumburg, IL 60173-4973 or online at www.asahq.org.

(**Table 4**) may require airway interventions. It is important that the anesthesia provider or, when the anesthesia team is not involved in the case, main proceduralist and, if any, the sedation provider make an adequate evaluation of the patient's airway and are aware of any potential problems in case any airway interventions become necessary (eg, in the case of hypoventilation or even apnea resulting in hypoxia because of the effect of a sedative, or episode of laryngospasm related to excessive airway secretions during upper endoscopy resulting in desaturation of oxygen level) so the team can be adequately prepared to protect patient safety.

There are several predictors of a "difficult airway":

- Predictors of difficult intubation[18,19]:
  - Higher Mallampati classification (III–IV)
  - Short thyromental distance (<3 finger breaths or 6 cm)
  - Limited neck range of motion
  - Shorter interincisor gap (<4 cm)
  - Class III upper-lip bite test (lower incisors cannot reach the upper lip)
  - Other factors, such as congenital syndromes that result in dysmorphic facial features, acromegaly, rheumatoid arthritis affecting cervical neck, temporomandibular joint dysfunction
- Predictors of difficult mask ventilation[20–23]:
  - Increased BMI
  - History of sleep apnea/snoring
  - Presence of beard
  - Lack of teeth
  - Age greater than 55 years
  - Mallampati class III–IV
  - Limited mandibular protrusion test
  - Male gender
  - Airway mass/tumor

If these features are present and sedation level deeper than minimal sedation/anxiolysis is needed for the procedure, involving the anesthesia provider team should be considered.

Table 4
Definition of general anesthesia and levels of sedation/analgesia

	Minimal Sedation Anxiolysis	Moderate Sedation/ Analgesia ("Conscious Sedation")	Deep Sedation/Analgesia	General Anesthesia
Responsiveness	Normal response to verbal stimulation	Purposeful response to verbal or tactile stimulation	Purposeful response following repeated or painful stimulation	Unarousable even with painful stimulus
Airway	Unaffected	No intervention required	Intervention may be required	Intervention often required
Spontaneous ventilation	Unaffected	Adequate	May be inadequate	Frequently inadequate
Cardiovascular function	Unaffected	Usually maintained	Usually maintained	May be impaired

Reflex withdrawal from a painful stimulus is NOT considered a purposeful response.

Excerpted from ASA, Continuum of Depth of Sedation: Definition of General Anesthesia and Levels of Sedation/Analgesia (Approved by the ASA House of Delegates on October 13, 1999, and last amended on October 23, 2019) of the American Society of Anesthesiologists. A copy of the full text can be obtained from ASA, 1061 American Lane Schaumburg, IL 60173-4973 or online at www.asahq.org.

ANESTHETIC MANAGEMENT

Type of anesthesia and level of sedation are chosen based on the type of procedure, specific requirements of the procedure, emergency/urgency of the procedure, and patient factors as described previously.

Conscious Sedation, Monitored Anesthesia Care, and General Anesthesia

In regard to the level of sedation, ASA has published descriptions of the continuum of depth of sedation (see **Table 4**). Of note, several endoscopic procedures are frequently performed under monitored anesthesia care (MAC). Although the term is often loosely used to describe anesthesia care involving no endotracheal intubation or laryngeal mask airway insertion, it refers to a specific anesthesia service performed by a qualified anesthesia provider and does not refer to a specific depth of sedation.[24] One of the indications for MAC includes "the need for deeper levels of analgesia and sedation than can be provided by moderate sedation (including potential conversion to a general or regional anesthetic)."[25] Also note that, contrary to common misconception, general anesthesia does not always involve airway intervention.

Conscious sedation versus monitored anesthesia care

Both upper and lower GI endoscopic procedures are routinely performed under moderate sedation ("conscious sedation") administered by a nonanesthesia provider and are well tolerated by patients. Common complaints include anxiety, discomfort/pain, and "waking up during the procedure." A detailed preprocedural discussion with the patient regarding the level of sedation, providing reassurance, and setting the appropriate expectations (eg, make the patient aware that they are not "going under" and some amount of recall is normal and expected) help mitigate such complaints and improve patient satisfaction. However, involving the anesthesia team for MAC should be considered in following situations:

- In operations whereby sedation level deeper than moderate will likely be required (also refer to Preanesthetic/Preprocedural Evaluations above; these include advanced procedures that are likely to have longer procedural times, those that require minimal patient movements during, or where the patient is not expected to tolerate the procedure without deeper level of sedation for reasons such as pain, severe anxiety, or tolerance to sedatives);
- Patients with complicated comorbidities and/or high ASA class (III–IV);
- Patients with known history of difficult airway or physical examination signs of difficult airway described above;
- Patients who are at high risk of aspiration but are not suitable for minimal sedation;
- Urgent or emergent cases.

The key is to thoroughly evaluate the needs of the scheduled procedure and its expected course as well as potential difficulties (if any) along with patient's history and physical examination findings. Performing such procedures under MAC allows delivery of appropriate level of sedation or general anesthesia to facilitate the operation. It also allows the team to be prepared for possible airway interventions and to decrease the risk of potential complications, such as prolonged hypoxia, pulmonary aspiration.

Endotracheal Intubation for Endoscopic Operations

Endotracheal intubation should be considered for patients who are at high risk of aspiration (eg, GERD, motility disorders such as achalasia, gastroparesis, gastric outlet obstruction, small bowel obstruction, upper GI bleeding, conditions that increase intraabdominal pressure such as large ascites, structural abnormalities such as Zenker's diverticulum), in certain complicated procedures, or in emergency situations for airway protection. A randomized controlled trial by Smith and colleagues[26] comparing general endotracheal anesthesia (GEA) versus MAC without endotracheal intubation in patients at high risk of sedation-related adverse events showed a significantly lower incidence of when GEA was used, without impacting procedure duration, success, recovery, or in-room time.

Several airway management techniques may be considered in patients with high risk of aspiration. These techniques include rapid sequence intubation (RSI) and awake fiberoptic intubation.

Rapid sequence intubation

Compared with typical induction and intubation, the RSI technique involves use of rapidly acting neuromuscular blocking agent (typically succinylcholine unless contraindicated, in which case a "rapid sequence dose" or a higher than usual intubating dose of nondepolarizing neuromuscular blocking agent is administered), omission of mask ventilation to decrease the risk of insufflating the stomach, and application of cricoid pressure (Sellick maneuver) during induction. The goal of RSI is to minimize the time between induction of anesthesia and securing of the airway with a cuffed endotracheal tube. Providers in the operating room are sometimes asked to assist anesthesia providers in applying cricoid pressure during RSI. Originally described by Sellick[27] nearly 60 years ago, cricoid pressure involves application of pressure at about 10 N (2.5 lbs) at the level of the cricoid ring while the patient is awake and 30 N after loss of consciousness to occlude the esophageal lumen.[28] Cricoid pressure should be applied at induction and should not be released until endotracheal intubation is confirmed (typically via appearance of end-tidal CO_2 on the ventilator or auscultation of bilateral breath sounds).

Awake fiberoptic intubation

During an awake intubation, endotracheal intubation is performed with the assistance of a fiberoptic bronchoscope while the patient is awake, spontaneously ventilating with intact protective airway reflexes. Topical anesthetics are administered to blunt gag reflex and to improve patient comfort and tolerance of the procedure. Sedatives and a low dose of intravenous anesthetics are also frequently administered, but careful titration is crucial to avoid apnea or blunting of the airway reflex because of deeper-than-intended level of sedation during the process.

Use of video laryngoscope

Video laryngoscopes are frequently used in conjunction with the above techniques. Literature suggests that there is a higher chance of successful intubation at first attempt when video laryngoscopes are used, especially in difficult airways.[29]

Furthermore, placement of a nasogastric tube and suctioning of the gastric contents should be considered in a patient with bowel obstruction before induction of anesthesia to decrease the gastric volume and risk of aspiration.

Monitoring

ASA has published guidelines for moderate procedural sedation and analgesia[30] as well as for sedation and analgesia by nonanesthesiologists.[31] The most recent guidelines for moderate procedural sedation (2018) recommend the following:

- Periodic (5-minute intervals) monitoring of patient's response to verbal commands

- Continuous monitoring of ventilatory function by qualitative observation, capnography, and pulse oximetry
- Presedation blood pressure
- Monitoring of blood pressure and heart rate at 5-minute intervals
- Electrocardiography in the case of patients with clinically significant cardiovascular disease
- Use of supplemental oxygen unless contraindicated

The presence of a trained individual other than the one performing the procedure is also recommended. Per American Society for Gastrointestinal Endoscopy guidelines for sedation and anesthesia in GI endoscopy,[32] providers of GI endoscopy should be trained to provide procedural sedation across the sedation continuum from minimal through moderate sedation as well as rescue skills in cases whereby the level of sedation is deeper than intended.

Performing Endoscopic Operations Under Anesthesia at an Ambulatory Surgery Center

Advanced endoscopic operations are often performed at hospital-based endoscopy units. The number of endoscopic operations scheduled at ambulatory surgery centers (ASCs) and ambulatory endoscopy centers (AECs) have been on the increase, and a prospective study in 2016 evaluated the safety profile of performing such procedures in an ASC. Mok and colleagues[33] showed that endoscopic retrograde cholangiopancreatography (ERCP) and endoscopic ultrasound (EUS) can be performed in a higher-risk population under the supervision of anesthesia in ASCs with an equivalent adverse event rate as inpatients.

In addition to meeting Centers for Medicare & Medicaid Services (CMS) standards for an ASC and being accredited, emergency equipment and medications should be readily available in the procedural area and maintained on a regular basis. The emergency equipment and medications includes advanced airway equipment, suction, positive pressure ventilation device, oxygen source, self-inflating hand resuscitator bag, medications including antagonists for benzodiazepines and opioids, and a defibrillator.[30,34,35] An individual trained in advanced cardiac life support (ACLS) should be immediately available as well. There should be a designated area and appropriately trained personnel to provide postanesthesia management.[36] An anesthesiologist responsible for the care will perform preanesthetic and postanesthetic assessments, and discharge from postanesthesia care unit (PACU) is a physician's responsibility.[36]

There are several aspects of performing endoscopic operations in an ambulatory setting that should be considered to ensure time- and cost-effective operation.

Location and organization

At the author's institution, preprocedural and postprocedural beds are located in the immediate vicinity of the procedural area. A patient who presents for an endoscopic operation is brought to a preprocedural room for intake, nursing assessments, and intravenous access placement; an anesthesiologist interviews the patient and completes preanesthetic assessment in this area before the operation. Once the procedure is completed, the patient is brought to a postanesthesia room until appropriate discharge criteria are met.[36] The anesthesiologist oversees postanesthesia care, evaluates the patient, and discusses any significant issues with the proceduralist, which ensures that appropriate postoperative care is provided. The proximity of the areas, efficient room turnover, and prompt identification of any preprocedural or postprocedural issues by appropriately trained personnel (eg, issues regarding NPO status, bowel preparation, postprocedural pain are immediately communicated to physicians by the nursing team) as well as immediate availability of the anesthesiologist result in an efficient unit with appropriate utilization of the time and resources.

Scheduling

An analysis performed by Tsai and colleagues[37] concluded that changing anesthesia block allocations in endoscopy can improve productivity and decrease opportunity-unused time. At the author's institution, it is determined by the proceduralist at the time of booking whether a patient should undergo his or her procedure under anesthesia or conscious sedation (without anesthesia providers). Anesthesia blocks are arranged in such a way that one endoscopist's procedures that need to be performed under anesthesia are scheduled in one room in a series. If there is a procedure room(s) designated for nonanesthesia cases, one proceduralist is typically scheduled in the room for the day with his or her patients along with a provider trained to administer conscious sedation. This arrangement improves time efficiency by minimizing wait and turnover times, as there is no need for proceduralists or anesthesia providers to switch between operating rooms throughout the day.

Anesthesia Care Team Model

An anesthesia care team includes both physicians and nonphysicians.[38] Typically, a care team consists of an anesthesiologist plus either a resident/fellow physician or an anesthetist. The term anesthetist refers to a registered nurse certified in anesthesia training program (CRNA) or a health professional who is certified in an anesthesiologist assistant program (CAA or AA). An anesthesiologist may medically direct 1 to 4 CRNAs concurrently. A team-based approach in the practice of anesthesiology ensures comprehensive perioperative management of patients: preanesthetic medical optimization, prescription of appropriate anesthetic plan by a trained physician and monitoring, postanesthetic evaluation and care. In an endoscopic operation suite where there are typically multiple scheduled cases, efficient case flow can be maintained by allowing immediate availability of the anesthesiologist to all phases of perioperative care (eg, the anesthesiologist is able to assess and optimize a patient in the preprocedure area, address any postoperative complications while personally participating in all demanding procedures of an anesthesia plan) while constant monitoring of an anesthetized patient is carried out by anesthetists or training physicians. As the process and demands of a GI endoscopic procedure are unique compared with a general surgical case, the anesthesia team should familiarize themselves with the scheduled procedure and patient's medical history to provide optimal care and minimize delays. Good communication between the endoscopist, anesthesiologist, and anesthetist plays a crucial role in improving time efficiency and productivity.

Postanesthesia Care

Any patients who receive general anesthesia or MAC should receive appropriate postanesthesia management. In most cases, this requires having a designated PACU with appropriately trained providers who can recognize any anesthetic complications (the design, equipment, and staffing of the PACU shall meet requirements of the facility's accrediting and licensing bodies[36]). PACU should be equipped with supplemental oxygen, suction, and basic monitors and have access to emergency equipment ("code cart" with advanced airway equipment and medications). Common issues that arise in PACU after an endoscopic procedure include pain (eg, abdominal discomfort related to insufflation, sore throat from either/both insertion of an endoscope or endotracheal intubation, if performed), nausea, hypoxemia from oversedation and hypoventilation or OSA, hypotension related to anesthetics, hypertension, emergence delirium, or confusion. Rarer complications such as cardiac arrythmias, may occur and are often related to the patient's medical history. Symptoms of procedural complication such as pneumoperitoneum, pneumothorax, gas embolism, and bowel perforation, may also be recognized in PACU if not noted immediately during the operation. Continual evaluation of the patient's condition in PACU is therefore essential.

SUMMARY

There is an increasing demand for endoscopic procedures in patients with complicated medical history. Many of these patients are considered to be "too high risk" for an open surgical operation, whereas a less-invasive endoscopic procedure may serve for both diagnostic and therapeutic purposes. Also, some of the advanced endoscopic operations need fine optimization that make conscious sedation inefficient or uncomfortable for patients. Performing these operations under anesthesia can facilitate the procedure by not only providing an optimal procedural condition but also allowing the endoscopist to focus on the procedural aspects while the anesthesia team manages the patient's airway, hemodynamics, depth of sedation, or general anesthesia. Advanced endoscopic procedures can be safely performed with anesthesia care in ambulatory settings as well (ASC and AEC), and attentive scheduling of cases can help improve efficiency and productivity. A thorough preanesthetic evaluation starting with history and physical examination with a focus on NPO status, ASA status, airway evaluations, and medical history that places the patient at high risk of aspiration should guide the decision on the type of sedation or anesthesia.

CLINICS CARE POINTS

- When performing preprocedural history and physical examination, evaluate for risk of aspiration and physical findings indicative of difficult airway. These factors should be considered in determining the appropriateness of conscious sedation.
- Endotracheal intubation should be strongly considered in patients with high risk of aspiration, as it may reduce incidence of adverse events without affecting procedural factors.
- Consider involving the anesthesia care team when a complex endoscopic procedure is to be performed in a patient with complicated medical history.
- When implementing anesthesia cases in an ambulatory surgery center/ambulatory endoscopy center, pay close attention to scheduling to improve time efficiency and productivity.

DISCLOSURE

The author has nothing to disclose.

REFERENCES

1. Barakat MT, et al. Escalating complexity of endoscopic retrograde cholangiopancreatography over the last decade with increasing reliance on advanced cannulation techniques. World J Gastroenterol 2020;26(41):6391–401.
2. Hwang JH, et al. GIE editorial board top 10 topics: advances in GI endoscopy in 2019. Gastrointest Endosc 2020;92(2):241–51.

3. Nagrebetsky A, et al. Growth of nonoperating room anesthesia care in the United States: a contemporary trends analysis. Anesth Analg 2017;124(4):1261–7.

4. Bhavani SS, Abdelmalak B. Nonoperating room anesthesia: anesthesia in the gastrointestinal suite. Anesthesiol Clin 2019;37(2):301–16.

5. Tetzlaff JE, Vargo JJ, Maurer W. Nonoperating room anesthesia for the gastrointestinal endoscopy suite. Anesthesiol Clin 2014;32(2):387–94.

6. Al-Awabdy B, Wilcox CM. Use of anesthesia on the rise in gastrointestinal endoscopy. World J Gastrointest Endosc 2013;5(1):1–5.

7. Predmore Z, et al. Anesthesia service use during outpatient gastroenterology procedures continued to increase from 2010 to 2013 and potentially discretionary spending remained high. Am J Gastroenterol 2017;112(2):297–302.

8. Shahrokh Iravani MF, Zojaji H, Azizi M, et al. Pedram Azimzadeh, Effect of general anesthesia during GI endoscopic procedures on patient satisfaction. Gastroenterol Hepatol From Bed Bench 2012;5(Suppl 1):S20–5.

9. Birk J, Bath RK. Is the anesthesiologist necessary in the endoscopy suite? A review of patients, payers and safety. Expert Rev Gastroenterol Hepatol 2015;9(7):883–5.

10. Singh H, et al. Propofol for sedation during colonoscopy. Cochrane Database Syst Rev 2008;(4):Cd006268.

11. Mayhew D, Mendonca V, Murthy BVS. A review of ASA physical status - historical perspectives and modern developments. Anaesthesia 2019;74(3):373–9.

12. Enestvedt BK, et al. Is the American Society of Anesthesiologists classification useful in risk stratification for endoscopic procedures? Gastrointest Endosc 2013;77(3):464–71.

13. Sharma VK, et al. A national study of cardiopulmonary unplanned events after GI endoscopy. Gastrointest Endosc 2007;66(1):27–34.

14. Curatolo C, et al. ASA physical status assignment by non-anesthesia providers: do surgeons consistently downgrade the ASA score preoperatively? J Clin Anesth 2017;38:123–8.

15. ASA. ASA Physical Status Classification System. (Approved by the ASA House of Delegates on October 15, 2014, and last amended on December 13, 2020). Available at: https://www.asahq.org/standards-and-guidelines/asa-physical-status-classification-system. Accessed December 13, 2020.

16. Green SM, Mason KP, Krauss BS. Pulmonary aspiration during procedural sedation: a comprehensive systematic review. Br J Anaesth 2017;118(3):344–54.

17. Practice guidelines for preoperative fasting and the use of pharmacologic agents to reduce the risk of pulmonary aspiration: application to healthy patients undergoing elective procedures: an updated report by the American Society of Anesthesiologists Task Force on preoperative fasting and the use of pharmacologic agents to reduce the risk of pulmonary aspiration. Anesthesiology 2017;126(3):376–93.

18. Sunanda Gupta RS. Dimpel Jain, Airway assessment predictors of difficult airway. Indian J Anaesthesia 2005;49(4):257.

19. Seo SH, et al. Predictors of difficult intubation defined by the intubation difficulty scale (IDS): predictive value of 7 airway assessment factors. Korean J Anesthesiol 2012;63(6):491–7.

20. El-Orbany M, Woehlck HJ. Difficult mask ventilation. Anesth Analgesia 2009;109(6):1870–80.

21. Kheterpal S, et al. Incidence and predictors of difficult and impossible mask ventilation. Anesthesiology 2006;105(5):885–91.

22. Langeron O, et al. Prediction of difficult mask ventilation. Anesthesiology 2000; 92(5):1229–36.
23. Yildiz TS, Solak M, Toker K. The incidence and risk factors of difficult mask ventilation. J Anesth 2005;19(1):7–11.
24. ASA. Continuum of depth of sedation: definition of general anesthesia and levels of sedation/analgesia. (Approved by the ASA House of Delegates on October 13, 1999, and last amended on October 23, 2019). Available at: https://www.asahq.org/standards-and-guidelines/continuum-of-depth-of-sedation-definition-of-general-anesthesia-and-levels-of-sedationanalgesia. Accessed December 1, 2020.
25. ASA. Position on monitored anesthesia care. (Approved by the House of Delegates on October 25, 2005, and last amended on October 17, 2018). Available at: https://www.asahq.org/standards-and-guidelines/position-on-monitored-anesthesia-care. Accessed December 1, 2020.
26. Smith ZL, et al. A randomized controlled trial evaluating general endotracheal anesthesia versus monitored anesthesia care and the incidence of sedation-related adverse events during ERCP in high-risk patients. Gastrointest Endosc 2019;89(4):855–62.
27. Sellick BA. Cricoid pressure to control regurgitation of stomach contents during induction of anaesthesia. Lancet 1961;2(7199):404–6.
28. Vanner RG, Asai T. Safe use of cricoid pressure. Anaesthesia 1999;54(1):1–3.
29. Russell TM, Hormis A. Should the glidescope video laryngoscope be used first line for all oral intubations or only in those with a difficult airway? A review of current literature. J Perioper Pract 2018;28(12):322–33.
30. Practice guidelines for moderate procedural sedation and analgesia 2018: a report by the American Society of Anesthesiologists Task Force on Moderate Procedural Sedation and Analgesia, the American Association of Oral and Maxillofacial Surgeons, American College of Radiology, American Dental Association, American Society of Dentist Anesthesiologists, and Society of Interventional Radiology. Anesthesiology 2018;128(3):437–79.
31. ASA Task Force on sedation and analgesia by non-anesthesiologists, practice guidelines for sedation and analgesia by non-anesthesiologists. Anesthesiology 2002;96(4):1004–17.
32. Early DS, et al. Guidelines for sedation and anesthesia in GI endoscopy. Gastrointest Endosc 2018;87(2):327–37.
33. Mok SR, et al. Therapeutic endoscopy can be performed safely in an ambulatory surgical center: a multicenter, prospective study. Diagn Ther Endosc 2016;2016: 7168280.
34. ASA. Guidelines for ambulatory anesthesia and surgery. (Approved by the ASA House of Delegates on October 15, 2003, last amended on October 22, 2008, and reaffirmed on October 17, 2018). Available at: https://www.asahq.org/standards-and-guidelines/guidelines-for-ambulatory-anesthesia-and-surgery. Accessed December 1, 2020.
35. ASA. Statement on nonoperating room anesthetizing locations. (Approved by the ASA House of Delegates on October 19, 1994, last amended on October 16, 2013, and reaffirmed on October 17, 2018). Available at: https://www.asahq.org/standards-and-guidelines/statement-on-nonoperating-room-anesthetizing-locations. Accessed December 1, 2020.
36. ASA. Standards for postanesthesia care. (Approved by the ASA House of Delegates on October 27, 2004, and last amended on October 23, 2019). Available at: https://www.asahq.org/standards-and-guidelines/standards-for-postanesthesia-care. Accessed December 1, 2020.

37. Tsai MH, et al. Changing anesthesia block allocations improves endoscopy suite efficiency. J Med Syst 2019;44(1):1.
38. ASA. Statement on the anesthesia care team. (Approved by the ASA House of Delegates on October 26, 1982 and last amended on October 23, 2019). Available at: https://www.asahq.org/standards-and-guidelines/position-on-monitored-anesthesia-care. Accessed December 1, 2020.

The Future of Endoscopic Operations After the Coronavirus Pandemic

Klaus Mergener, MD, PhD, MBA

KEYWORDS

- Coronavirus • COVID-19 pandemic • Gastroenterology • GI endoscopy
- Practice management

KEY POINTS

- Modern GI practices have a high overhead structure and are thus vulnerable to sudden interruptions in cash flow.
- Professional management and constant vigilance are necessary to respond quickly to new developments and adapt expense and revenue structures as needed.
- Procedure backlogs from COVID shutdowns have resulted in delayed GI care that needs to be addressed in a structured fashion, with higher-risk patients prioritized for examinations.
- The pandemic accelerated the implementation of telemedicine programs, and these services will continue to be used in the postpandemic era.
- A crisis presents challenges but also opportunities, and the sense of accomplishment from having navigated this crisis will result in a strong culture of teamwork.

INTRODUCTION

The coronavirus disease 2019 (COVID-19) pandemic represents an unprecedented global health crisis that has challenged GI practices and endoscopy operations in major and unforeseen ways. As of March 1, 2021, there were 115 million confirmed cases of COVID-19 and more than 2.5 million deaths globally, with almost 30 million cases and more than 527,000 deaths in the United States alone.[1]

Rapidly implemented global shutdowns of everyday life and business, including medical operations, resulted in sudden delays in our ability to diagnose and treat GI illnesses and perform cancer screening. As the country is moving toward a full reopening supported by rapidly evolving vaccination programs and scientific discoveries related to the prevention and management of COVID-19, medical practices are wrestling with the challenge of a complete retooling of their operations with the goal of

Division of Gastroenterology, University of Washington, 1917 Warren Avenue North, Seattle, WA 98109, USA
E-mail address: klausmergener@aol.com
Twitter: @kmergener (K.M.)

Gastrointest Endoscopy Clin N Am 31 (2021) 773–785
https://doi.org/10.1016/j.giec.2021.05.012
1052-5157/21/

giendo.theclinics.com

quickly returning to providing high-quality care to large numbers of patients safely and effectively.

At the same time, assessment has begun of the long-term impact that the current pandemic may have on future practice operations: What will postpandemic GI care look like, and how soon will we get there? Will we return to prepandemic operations in all aspects of our work, or will some elements of GI practice be changed forever? If so, what are those elements, and what are the implications for GI leaders as they look to position their groups for continued success? This chapter provides an overview of the impact of the pandemic on US-based GI practices and discusses some key "lessons learned" that may affect future operations.

THE PREPANDEMIC STATE OF GI PRACTICE

Before discussing the ongoing impact of COVID-19 on GI groups and endoscopy operations, it is useful to briefly take stock of the recent history and challenges encountered by GI practices prior to 2020.

Gastroenterologists have enjoyed great success due to the large burden of GI disease and thus high demand for GI services. In our health care system, with its predominantly fee-for-service reimbursement, procedural specialties have fared well economically. Still, there have been considerable and mounting challenges to the current GI practice model[2]: Reimbursement for endoscopic procedures has declined significantly in recent years while practice costs have continued to skyrocket. Many primary care providers have become employed by payers or large health systems, thereby affecting patient referral patterns for specialty services. Hospital and payer consolidation has resulted in a rapidly changing landscape where small practices often lose leverage in contract negotiations. Disruptive technologies such as nonendoscopic tests for cancer screening and advances in radiology have the potential to further challenge a specialty that is now heavily reliant on revenue from endoscopic procedures.

At the same time, gastroenterologists have been resilient in meeting current challenges. Moving many endoscopic services from the hospital to physician-owned ambulatory endoscopy centers has allowed physicians to increase efficiencies and capture income from facility fees. Adding ancillary revenue streams such as pathology, anesthesia services, infusion, and imaging centers has allowed some groups to compensate for the continued decline in professional fees.[2]

As a result, the prepandemic GI practice had evolved from a low-overhead hospital-based operation to a high-overhead business with high capital investments and thus a significant dependence on efficient, high-throughput endoscopy services to generate constant cash flow in support of its cost structure. While this potential vulnerability was not lost on astute practice managers, there was no reason to believe that smoothly running endoscopy services would experience a sudden interruption and downturn in procedure volumes.

THE COVID-19 PANDEMIC

Such was the situation in late December 2019 when the first report arrived at the World Health Organization (WHO) from Wuhan, China, about a new type of pneumonia of unknown cause.[3] The ensuing weeks and months brought the most rapid progress of science ever accomplished in the history of infectious diseases: The responsible agent for COVID-19 was identified as a novel beta-coronavirus, now termed severe acute respiratory syndrome coronavirus 2 (SARS-CoV-2).[4] The virus was isolated on January 7, the full genome sequence was published on January 10, and the first fully validated polymerase chain reaction (PCR) testing protocol was shared with the WHO on January 13, 2020. Since then, the molecular structure of this virus has been determined, PCR, antigen, and antibody tests have been developed, and numerous studies have been performed to elucidate the mechanism of viral transmission, the immunologic response of the host, disease characteristics, treatment options, and vaccine development. Several key findings from this research provide important insights into the anticipated impact of COVID-19 on GI practices and endoscopic operations going forward.[4,5]

Virus Structure and Transmission

The genetic sequence and structure of SARS-Co-V-2 are similar to those of other human coronaviruses. A lipid bilayer envelope makes the virus particle susceptible to regular detergents, thereby facilitating virus deactivation with standard cleaning procedures such as those used during regular endoscope reprocessing. The spike glycoprotein (S-protein) is embedded in the viral envelope and mediates host cell binding and entry. S-protein has been identified as the main target in current vaccine development efforts,[6] and monoclonal anti-S antibodies have been produced as one of the first therapeutic agents to combat COVID-19 illness.[7] The 30 kb single-strand RNA genome of SARS-CoV-2 encodes several other structural and nonstructural proteins, including a replication proofreading apparatus. While this might be expected to reduce the rate of virus mutations compared with other RNA viruses, there have been numerous reports in recent months of emerging virus variants that appear to confer higher transmissibility.[8] The full impact of these mutations on the epidemiology of COVID-19 and the effectiveness of vaccination programs remains incompletely understood, but this will be a major determinant of what GI practice operations will look like in the near to medium term.

SARS-CoV-2 infects epithelial cells in the respiratory and GI tracts and possibly other target cells. The incubation period ranges from 2 to 14 days, and symptomatic individuals are most contagious immediately before and within the first 5 days of symptom onset with a rapid decline of viral load thereafter.[9] A key determinant of the high transmissibility is that an estimated 40% to 50% of all COVID-19 infections are transmitted by individuals who are either presymptomatic or remain entirely asymptomatic during the course of their own infection.[10,11] This has important implications for the implementation of safety measures in the endoscopy unit because simple screening for COVID-19 symptoms will miss a large percentage of SARS-CoV-2 carriers. Virus transmission occurs at close range (within 2 m) via respiratory droplets expelled during coughing or sneezing but also via aerosol transmission, that is, microdroplets small enough to remain suspended in the air for 30 minutes or longer and expose individuals at distances beyond 2 m, often in poorly ventilated indoor settings without sufficient air exchange.[12] Infection via contaminated surfaces appears to play only a minor role, and the relative contributions of these different modalities are not fully known at present.[13] The role of fecal–oral transmission received considerable attention during the early stages of the pandemic but appears to be minimal if it occurs at all.[14,15] Although SARS-CoV-2 infects GI epithelial cells, and viral RNA can be identified in stool specimens via PCR testing, studies using viral culture have not consistently identified infectious particles in stool, and no credible reports exist in the English literature of clinically relevant fecal–oral transmission.

Propagation of the Pandemic and Initial Impact on Endoscopy Centers

Since its initial appearance in late 2019, COVID-19 has spread around the globe at an alarming pace. The first US case was reported in a Washington state resident who returned from Wuhan, China, on January 15, 2020. On January 31, 2020, WHO issued a global health emergency, and on March 11, WHO declared COVID-19 a pandemic. With cases rising rapidly, travel restrictions, business shutdowns, and stay-at-home orders followed within a few days. By the end of March 2020, endoscopy volumes for elective procedures had fallen to less than 10% of baseline volumes.[16–18]

At that point, endoscopy unit managers were confronted with a sudden and profound decrease in cash flow for these very cash-dependent operations. Strategies had to be developed quickly to (1) reduce expenses and (2) repair revenues. For the rapid reduction of expenses, the main cost drivers had to be identified and addressed: (1) staff costs needed to be reduced via layoffs and furloughs; (2) accounts payable such as rent and other contracts needed to be renegotiated as much as feasible; and (3) efforts to reduce operational costs/waste needed to be intensified. Revenue repair focused on the following items: (1) rapid implementation of telehealth capabilities, including training of patients and staff on IT platforms; (2) procurement of sufficient personal protective equipment (PPE) and retooling of workflows in the endoscopy center to allow at least partial resumption of elective operations as soon as state regulations allowed; (3) development of communication tools to (a) inform patients of the steps taken to maintain a safe environment in GI practice and endoscopy unit and (b) to keep staff up to date on the rapid implementation of these changes.

Since April 2020, the pandemic has progressed in a typical manner through phases of deceleration and acceleration. On April 7, daily case numbers reached the first peak of 35,000 before decreasing and then rising again to well over 80,000 cases per day in late July.[1] Another decrease was followed by an even larger third wave that peaked at more than 250,000 daily cases in early January 2021. At the time of this writing in March 2021, daily case numbers have again decreased and leveled off at a still concerningly high trough level of 45,000 to 50,000/d, with the direction of the next trend yet to be determined. Significant variability of this dynamic from state to state and the lack of a standardized federal approach to reopening and shutdown orders have resulted in a varied approach to and timing of reopening of endoscopy centers depending on their geographic location and local circumstances. At the 1-year mark of the COVID-19 pandemic on March 10, 2021, there is hope that the end of the pandemic can be reached by the end of summer 2021, mainly thanks to the rollout of a comprehensive vaccination program that has now begun.[19]

The Promise of COVID Vaccines

Initial COVID containment efforts focused on nonpharmacologic interventions to include social distancing, contact tracing, and isolation, the use of personal protective equipment (PPE) to include face masks, and handwashing and environmental cleaning. These efforts have now been significantly augmented by the development, approval, and rollout of COVID-19 vaccinations. Vaccines typically require years of research and testing before reaching clinical practice, but in early 2020, almost immediately after the identification of the molecular virology of SARS-CoV-2, scientists embarked on a race to produce safe and effective coronavirus vaccines in record time. By fall 2020, more than 150 vaccine candidates were in various stages of development.[6,20]

In the United States, 3 vaccines have now received emergency use authorization from the Food and Drug Administration.[21] While storage requirements and the number of necessary inoculations vary between products, all 3 vaccines result in a humoral and T-cell-mediated immune response against epitopes of the viral S-protein. Clinical trials to date have shown surprisingly high efficacy rates upwards of 85% to 94% for all 3 products,[22] with "efficacy" defined as a reduction in the rate of acquiring severe

COVID-19 disease. Importantly, and relevant to the risk of vaccinated individuals to still carry and transmit SARS-CoV-2 virus in endoscopy units, there is now emerging evidence that vaccinations also result in a marked decrease in viral load of up to 20-fold and therefore a projected lower risk of infection transmission.[23,24] While many details remain to be worked out, including the duration of protective immunity after vaccination and thus the need for and timing of possible future booster immunizations, the more immediate hope relates to continuing with rapid vaccine administration, currently occurring at a rate of 2 million individuals per day in the United States,[25] in order to reach "herd immunity." This term refers to the percentage of a population that must acquire immunity to an infectious agent in order for the transmission of the agent to slow and eventually seize. In the case of SARS-CoV-2, many experts predict that "herd immunity" requires that at least 70% of the population has become immune to COVID-19 through either vaccination or natural infection.[26] It is important to note that the "end of the COVID-19 pandemic" should not be envisioned as flipping a switch but rather as a stepwise process whereby, after reaching herd immunity, non-pharmacologic interventions to prevent COVID-19 transmission may be gradually lifted but could remain in effect in some areas or be implemented again at a later time depending on local disease prevalence. In addition, because not all individuals will have received or agreed to receive COVID vaccination, endoscopy units may still have to consider testing protocols or contact safety measures in nonvaccinated individuals in the event of persistently high case numbers in some geographic areas.

INITIAL REOPENING STRATEGIES AND SHORT-TERM IMPACT ON ENDOSCOPY OPERATIONS

The rapid spread of the COVID-19 pandemic in spring 2020 forced GI practice leaders to quickly develop contingency plans for their operations in order to provide uninterrupted GI care wherever feasible, maintain the solvency of the practice, and plan for a return to prepandemic patient volumes as soon as possible.[17,27] Many of these strategies have a budgetary impact, as they either require a financial investment or result in lower endoscopy unit throughput. Planning for the gradual resumption of services began during the first pandemic wave and was periodically updated as states proceeded through reopening and repeated shutdown mandates over the course of the pandemic. The American Society for Gastrointestinal Endoscopy (ASGE)[28] and several other professional organizations have produced guidance documents to provide gastroenterologists with recommendations to employ to mitigate infection risk and optimize endoscopy operations under these unique circumstances.[29–31]

Changes in Workflow

Creating a safe environment in the endoscopy unit for patients, staff, and providers should always remain the top priority for GI leaders. Preprocedure screening now includes a COVID symptom questionnaire, which should be mandatory for patients before any endoscopy and for staff at the beginning of each workday.[28] Symptom screening will miss asymptomatic and presymptomatic carriers, but positive responses in these questionnaires should prompt removal of the individual from care areas and self-quarantine or hospital referral as needed. Many practices have now included similar COVID-related questions in the postprocedure questionnaires typically used to assess patient satisfaction. Such questionnaires can be distributed and returned before and after endoscopy appointments, avoiding delays in workflows on the day of the procedure. Lobby, admittance area, and recovery bay capacities, as well as foot traffic, in the endoscopy center have been altered to accommodate the need for physical distancing, including fewer chairs in waiting areas, physical barriers (eg, plexiglass partitions) where physical distancing cannot be accomplished, and the implementation of unidirectional flow through the endoscopy unit wherever possible. Wearing a face mask that covers both mouth and nose has become mandatory for all patients, providers, and staff at all times, as it has been clearly shown to reduce the risk of COVID transmission.[32] A significant investment of both time and money is required for training patients and staff on the unit's COVID-19 protocols including new workflows, proper hand hygiene and disinfection procedures, timing of patient arrivals, discharge procedures, pickup by family members, etc.[28] Preprocedure office visits, generally poorly compensated but sometimes necessary in higher-risk patients referred for open-access procedures, are now commonly conducted via telemedicine.

Changes in the Endoscopy Room

Significant changes have been implemented in the endoscopy room as well in an attempt to minimize the risk of infection transmission.[33] All members of the endoscopy team need to wear a full set of PPE (gown, gloves, hair cover, eye protection), and the appropriate donning and doffing of PPE requires diligent training and frequent reinforcement.[28] Although the evidence supporting the use of a face mask to reduce the risk of infection is irrefutable, the decision regarding the choice of mask for endoscopy team members—specifically, whether to use N95 respirators versus regular surgical masks in the procedure room—is complex and not well supported by high-quality evidence. Some studies have shown surgical masks to be noninferior to N95 respirators in the prevention of viral infections like influenza,[34] but a recent systematic review and meta-analysis showed a benefit in using N95 respirators over standard masks in protecting health care workers from SARS-CoV-1.[35] While these devices are more costly than regular surgical masks, they should therefore be strongly considered (assuming no supply shortage) for team members in the endoscopy room, given that upper endoscopies are known to generate aerosols. While the advantage of N95 masks over surgical masks will diminish with decreasing prevalence of SARS-CoV-2, endoscopy units are well advised to err on the side of safety until vaccination efforts and testing can provide assurance of negligible COVID risk.

Some authors have suggested additional time for room aeration between individual endoscopic procedures even in ambulatory endoscopy settings, a recommendation that remains a topic of intense debate and has not been widely adopted. The rationale for increasing the number of air exchanges between cases rests on the notion of SARS-CoV-2 being transmitted via aerosols and thus remaining airborne for prolonged periods in indoor settings with poor ventilation. ASGE guidance notes that "rooms lacking negative pressure benefit from additional aeration time for adequate clearance of droplets/aerosols,"[28] and some authors have suggested that this extra time between procedures should be as long as 30 to 60 minutes per case, an approach that is economically prohibitive for busy endoscopy units. In the absence of definitive scientific evidence specific to the endoscopy unit, different centers have taken very different approaches, and more studies are required to inform these decisions. Because of the high susceptibility of coronaviruses to standard disinfectant solutions, no changes are recommended to established reprocessing procedures for endoscopes and accessories.[26] While infection transmission via contaminated surfaces may play a comparatively minor role in the spread of SARS-CoV-2, professional organizations recommend deep cleaning of high-touch surfaces in procedure rooms after each case.[28,29] No changes are recommended to "terminal cleaning" procedures for cleaning and disinfecting the endoscopy unit at the end of the day.[36]

Testing Strategies

Because asymptomatic SARS-CoV-2 infections are a frequent source for transmission, a preprocedure symptom-screen of all individuals presenting for endoscopy is insufficient to eliminate the risk of infection transmission in the endoscopy suite. Ideally, efforts to mitigate this risk require all patients (and staff) to demonstrate either the presence of convalescent antibodies to SARS-CoV-2 or a negative molecular test within 48 hours of a scheduled procedure (or in the case of staff, with some regularity—eg, weekly). Many endoscopy units have implemented a universal testing strategy for patients, especially because the cost of testing is currently borne by government agencies in most states. Performing such a test close to the date of a procedure is important to avoid a negative test result during the early incubation period with subsequent high viral loads at the time of the procedure. While a well-timed universal testing strategy may be desirable, several obstacles have made widespread implementation of such an approach difficult. First, sufficient test capacities were not available during the early stages of the pandemic, and reports persist of periodic test shortages in some geographic areas. Second, test results need to be available at the time of the procedure, as cancellations will result in a significant number of unused endoscopy slots and thus considerable inefficiencies. In addition, test accuracies are not perfect. The Infectious Diseases Society of America suggests against universal testing when PPE is readily available, noting significant rates of false-negative tests and thus lower negative predictive value in areas of high disease prevalence.[37] Testing is favored if PPE is limited. The American Gastroenterological Association has published a detailed decision-making guide related to preprocedure testing, taking into account the test used, prevalence of the disease, and several other factors.[38] While this guide provides a detailed framework for decision-making, its algorithm is complex, and its application in everyday GI practice is therefore somewhat limited. With the increasing availability of point-of-care (POC) antigen tests and the development of new rapid turnaround molecular tests, and with the pandemic beginning to recede, the approach to preprocedure testing can be expected to undergo further changes. It appears likely that testing will eventually be employed in a more focused and targeted manner—for example, POC testing for individuals who are unable to produce proof of up-to-date vaccination or immunity to SARS-CoV-2.[39]

LONG-TERM IMPACT OF COVID-19 ON ENDOSCOPY OPERATIONS
Macroeconomic Considerations

The COVID-19 pandemic has led to record job losses. In April and May 2020 alone, more than 36 million Americans filed for unemployment benefits, levels not seen since the Great Depression.[40] While some unemployed individuals will have switched to an employed spouse's coverage, gotten on a parent's plan, or stayed covered by their previous employer through a COBRA package, many likely turned to coverage through health insurance exchanges, got on a Medicaid plan, or became uninsured. The end result of these shifts in the insurance market is projected to be an overall increase in the percentage of individuals who lose coverage or have to switch to insurance products that reimburse providers at lower rates for some services. What's more, financial hardships encountered during the pandemic may motivate people to postpone elective medical services such as screening exams or forgo them altogether, resulting in decreased practice revenues.

The federal government has enacted several pieces of legislation to provide relief to individuals and corporations affected by the COVID-19 pandemic. These provisions have been largely financed through borrowing, thereby increasing the US national debt. While these interventions were thought to be necessary to stimulate the economy and avoid a depression, the resulting increase in the national debt will put additional pressure on future annual budgets, including allocations for Medicare, Medicaid, and other health insurance programs. The prepandemic changes related to decreasing reimbursements for physician and facility services can therefore be expected to accelerate further. At the same time, costs will continue to increase. While innovations in care delivery or new endoscopic techniques or technologies may result in as yet unpredictable paradigm shifts and open new opportunities for GI endoscopists, the more immediate change will relate to the need to manage ever-decreasing profit margins. Hospitals and health systems have some ability to navigate this situation by shifting costs among their diversified services or pursuing further consolidation to gain negotiating clout and demand higher pricing. On the other hand, single-specialty GI groups have only limited ways to respond. They will need to intensify prepandemic efforts to contain costs, reduce waste and optimize efficiencies.[2] Paradoxically, practices that entered the pandemic year with suboptimal management and a low efficiency/high-cost structure may be expected to have the most room for improvement, provided that they recognize the need to quickly adopt professional management. One approach to cost containment relates to sharing resources across a larger organization, that is, merging with other GI practices. This trend had already begun prior to the pandemic and was partially fueled by private equity-funded practice roll-up models. It is anticipated that these mergers into ever larger, often multistate practices will continue and that other partners, such as payers and/or health systems, will also demonstrate an increasing interest in practice partnerships or opportunities to acquire GI practices outright. As was the case before COVID-19, there will not be a "one-size-fits-all" solution, and the best way forward for an individual practice will vary by region and market.[2]

Minimizing the Impact of Delayed GI Care

One critically important issue with long-term impact relates to the procedure backlog that has accumulated as a result of endoscopy center shutdowns. Colonoscopy is the most commonly performed GI endoscopy procedure, and its widespread use has been a major factor in the decline of colorectal cancer (CRC) in this country.[41] It is well documented that the risk of being diagnosed with CRC in general, and with advanced-stage CRC in particular, increases significantly if screening is delayed or is not completed in a timely manner after an initial positive stool test.[42–44] For example, Corley and colleagues[45] reported a 3.2-fold increase in CRC detected in fecal immunochemistry test (FIT)-positive patients when colonoscopy was delayed for more than 12 months. Modeling studies to estimate the potential impact of COVID-19-related disruptions to screening on CRC incidence and mortality have found that this disruption will have a marked and prolonged impact on CRC incidence and deaths between 2020 and 2050 attributable to missed screening.[46] Early reports of "real-world data" match the near-term predictions from these modeling studies. Using data sets from the National Health Service in England, Morris and colleagues[47] calculated a relative reduction of 22% in the number of CRC cases detected and referred for treatment in that country for the April to October 2020 time frame compared with the prior year.

With endoscopy units shut down for several weeks in 2020, some practices have accumulated procedure backlogs of several thousand procedures. It is crucial for these practices to explore ways to increase procedure capacities, for example, by extending work hours or offering weekend endoscopy times. Higher-risk patients, such as those with symptoms or a positive FIT test should be prioritized to minimize the risk of delayed cancer diagnoses. Efforts need to be increased to minimize vacant procedure slots due to last-minute cancellations or poor colon preparation and to avoid nonindicated procedures in order to preserve valuable procedure time for examinations on individuals with a higher risk of harboring GI pathology. Importantly, because patients may still be reluctant to return to medical facilities because they may perceive a continued high risk of contracting COVID-19, enhanced communication efforts are necessary to inform patients and referring providers of the safety of GI endoscopic services and the benefits of undergoing potentially life-saving procedures. Ongoing monitoring of screening participation rates will demonstrate the effects of changing patient behaviors and will identify needs for further patient education. Previous studies have shown that mass media campaigns can improve screening participation, have positive effects on long-term health impacts, and are highly cost-effective.[48]

The Role of Telemedicine

The pandemic accelerated the implementation of telemedicine programs by many years.[49] Before COVID-19, most practices had barely begun experimenting with virtual visits, and most payers provided very low reimbursement rates for these services, if they paid at all. When telehealth in a typical practice suddenly grew from a few visits to many thousand visits per month, physicians, patients, and payers became increasingly aware of its significant benefits. Patients appreciate the option of a virtual visit, especially those individuals who live far away or have mobility issues. Physicians can more easily conduct interactions with patients who do not always require physical examinations—for example, follow-up discussions after procedures or certain preprocedure screening assessments.[50] Additional services such as professional translators can be provided with greater ease in the virtual world. Provided that reimbursement for such virtual visits will remain adequate, it can be anticipated that a significant percentage of physician–patient visits will continue to be conducted via telemedicine. Practices are therefore well advised to continue to invest in their IT infrastructures. The leap to telemedicine in spring 2020 was fast-tracked and could not always include the level of "at-the-elbow" support that is typically employed for this level of change. Practices will need to continue to optimize workflows and staff and provider training to provide patients with the best possible experience in these virtual encounters.

Pandemic Disruption as an Opportunity

Winston Churchill is credited with the quote "Never let a good crisis go to waste."[51] For GI groups, the COVID-19 pandemic of 2020–2021 was an unprecedented crisis that challenged all aspects of practice operations in unforeseen ways and brought some practices to the brink of insolvency. At the same time, after an initial phase of stress and struggle, the majority of GI practices have been able to pivot and adjust to the new realities, often with a massive team effort. Going forward, this should create a sense of shared mission and be reflected on by the entire team as a proud accomplishment. The most successful groups will have used this crisis to question restrictive routines and identify opportunities for creative change and innovation, an effort that may well leave them better positioned for the challenges of the future.

There are valuable lessons to be drawn from the pandemic: First, despite being well-positioned and in demand, our specialty is not immune to sudden and unexpected calamities. While COVID-19 represents the first global pandemic of our professional careers, it may not be the last. As noted in a recent review by Morens and Fauci,[52] our modern way of life, with increased global travel, crowded cities, and a changing environment, promotes the emergence of new infectious diseases and lays the foundation for rapid global spread. Practices should continue to expect the unexpected, remain on alert, and invest in professional management and an infrastructure that allows them to respond rapidly to new developments. Second, the basic tenets of practice management hold as true in calm as they do in crisis. Groups that enter a difficult period with a solid organizational infrastructure and sound financial health are likely to fare better than those who fail to continuously improve and optimize their operations. A solid foundation is most useful in times of earthquake. Third, and most importantly, although GI represents a specialty with a strong procedural focus, and the modern endoscopy unit is geared toward throughput and efficiency, the pandemic has provided a powerful reminder that at its core, GI endoscopy, and the entire practice of gastroenterology, is a team sport. GI leaders are well advised to invest in their staff at all levels of the organization, creating a sense of coherence and shared mission and a culture of teamwork. The most successful GI practices are taking great care of people, and they do so in large part by taking care of the people who take care of people! With these learnings incorporated into the postpandemic GI practice, the future of our specialty continues to be bright!

CLINICS CARE POINTS

- Continue to monitor and follow GI society guidelines for changes in practice workflows and endoscopic operations during the COVID pandemic to keep patients and staff safe.
- Prioritize higher-risk patients and develop additional procedure capacities to quickly reduce procedure backlogs and avoid long waiting times for patients with potential significant GI diseases.
- Invest in IT and telemedicine capabilities and continue to offer this service to patients postpandemic to support timely medical care.

DISCLOSURE

The author has nothing to disclose.

REFERENCES

1. Worldometer COVID-19 tracker. Available at: https://www.worldometers.info/. Accessed March 1, 2021.
2. Mergener K. Impact of health care reform on the independent GI practice. Gastrointest Endosc Clin N Am 2012;22(1):15–27.
3. Zhu N, Zhang D, Wang W, et al. A novel coronavirus from patients with pneumonia in China, 2019. N Engl J Med 2020;382:727–33.
4. Cevik M, Kuppalli K, Kindrachuk J, et al. Virology, transmission, and pathogenesis of SARS-CoV-2. BMJ 2020;371:m3862.
5. Hu B, Guo H, Zhou P, et al. Characteristics of SARS-CoV-2 and COVID-19. Nat Rev Microbiol 2021;19:141–54.
6. Krammer F. SARS-CoV-2 vaccines in development. Nature 2020;586:516–27.
7. Cohen MS. Monoclonal antibodies to disrupt progression of early COVID-19 infection. N Engl J Med 2021;384:289–91.
8. Baric RS. Emergence of a highly fit SARS-CoV-2 variant. N Engl J Med 2020;383: 2684–6.
9. Meyerowitz EA, Richterman A, Gandhi RT, et al. Transmission of SARS-CoV-2: a review of viral, host and environmental factors. Ann Intern Med 2021;174:69–79.

10. Buitrago-Garcia D, Egli-Gany D, Counotte MJ, et al. Occurrence and transmission potential of asymptomatic and presymptomatic SARS-CoV-2 infections: a living systematic review and meta-analysis. PLoS Med 2020;17(9):e1003346.

11. Meyerowitz EA, Richterman A, Bogoch II, et al. Towards an accurate and systematic characterisation of persistently asymptomatic infection with SARS-CoV-2. Lancet Infect Dis 2020;21(6):e163–9.

12. Leung NHL, Chu DKW, Shiu EYC, et al. Respiratory virus shedding in exhaled breath and efficacy of face masks. Nat Med 2020;26(5):676–80.

13. Kissler SM, Tedijanto C, Goldstein E, et al. Projecting the transmission dynamics of SARS-CoV-2 through the postpandemic period. Science 2020;368:860–8.

14. Gu J, Han B, Wang J. COVID-19: gastrointestinal manifestations and potential fecal-oral transmission. Gastroenterology 2020;158:1518–9.

15. Repici A, Aragona G, Cengia G, et al. Low risk of COVID-19 transmission in GI endoscopy. Gut 2020;69:1925–7.

16. Parasa S, Reddy N, Faigel DO, et al. Global impact of the COVID-19 pandemic on endoscopy: an international survey of 252 centers from 55 countries. Gastroenterology 2020;159:1579–81.

17. Forbes N, Smith ZL, Spitzer RL, et al. Changes in gastroenterology and endoscopy practices in response to the COVID-19 pandemic: results from a North American survey. Gastroenterology 2020;159:772–4.e13.

18. Repici A, Pace F, Gabbiadini R, et al. Endoscopy units and the coronavirus disease 2019 outbreak: a multicenter experience from Italy. Gastroenterology 2020; 159:363–6.

19. Available at: https://news.harvard.edu/gazette/story/2020/12/anthony-fauci-offers-a-timeline-for-ending-covid-19-pandemic/. Accessed March 7, 2021.

20. Krammer F. Pandemic vaccines: how are we going to be better prepared next time? Med 2020;1:28–32.

21. Available at: https://www.fda.gov/emergency-preparedness-and-response/coronavirus-disease-2019-covid-19/covid-19-vaccines. Accessed March 4, 2021.

22. Forni G, Mantovani A. COVID-19 vaccines: where we stand and challenges ahead. Cell Death Differ 2021;28:626–39.

23. Levine-Tiefenbrun M, Yelin I, Katz R, et al. Decreased SARS-CoV-2 viral load following vaccination. MedRxiv 2021. https://doi.org/10.1101/2021.02.06. 21251283.

24. Petter E, Mor O, Zuckerman N, et al. Initial real-world evidence for lower viral load of individuals who have been vaccinated by BNT162b2. MedRxiv 2021. https://doi.org/10.1101/2021.02.08.21251329.

25. Available at: https://www.nytimes.com/interactive/2020/us/covid-19-vaccine-doses. html. Accessed March 8, 2021.

26. Omer SB, Yildirim I, Forman HP. Herd immunity and implications for SARS-CoV-2 control. JAMA 2020;324:2095–6.

27. Repici A, Maselli R, Colombo M, et al. Coronavirus (COVID-19) outbreak: what the department of endoscopy should know. Gastrointest Endosc 2020;92:192–7.

28. American Society for Gastrointestinal Endoscopy. Guidance for resuming GI endoscopy and practice operations after the COVID-19 pandemic. Gastrointest Endosc 2020;92:743–7.

29. British Society of Gastroenterology. Endoscopy activity and COVID-19: British Society of Gastroenterology and Joint Advisory Group Guidance 2020. Available at: https://www.bsg.org.uk/covid-19-advice/endoscopy-activity-and-covid-19-bsg-and-jag-guidance/. Accessed March 7, 2021.

30. Gralnek IM, Hassan C, Beilenhoff U, et al. ESGE and ESGENA position statement on gastrointestinal endoscopy and the COVID-19 pandemic. Endoscopy 2020; 52:483–90.

31. American Society for Gastrointestinal Endoscopy. Gastroenterology professional society guidance on endoscopic procedures during the COVID-19 pandemic 2020. Available at: https://www.asge.org/home/resources/key-resources/covid-19-asge-updates-for-members/gastroenterology-professional-society-guidance-on-endoscopic-procedures-during-the-covid-19-pandemic. Accessed March 7, 2021.

32. Chu DK, Akl EA, Duda S, et al. Physical distancing, face masks, and eye protection to prevent person-to-person transmission of SARS-CoV-2 and prevent COVID-19: a systematic review and meta-analysis. Lancet 2020;395:1973–87.

33. Cennamo V, Bassi M, Landi S, et al. Redesign of a GI endoscopy unit during the COVID-19 emergency: a practical model. Dig Liver Dis 2020;52:1178–87.

34. Long Y, Hu T, Liu L, et al. Effectiveness of N95 respirators versus surgical masks against influenza: a systematic review and meta-analysis. J Evid Based Med 2020;13:93–101.

35. Offeddu V, Yung CF, Low MSF, et al. Effectiveness of masks and respirators against respiratory infections in healthcare workers: a systematic review and meta-analysis. Clin Infect Dis 2017;65:1934–42.

36. Petersen BT, Cohen J, Hambrick RD, et al. Multisociety guideline on reprocessing flexible GI endoscopes: 2016 update. Gastrointest Endosc 2017;8:282–94.

37. IDSA guidelines on the diagnosis of COVID-19: molecular diagnostic testing. Available at: https://www.idsociety.org/COVID19guidelines/dx. Accessed March 1, 2021.

38. Sultan S, Siddique SM, Altayar O, et al. AGA Institute rapid review and recommendations on the role of pre-procedure SARS-CoV-2 testing and endoscopy. Gastroenterol 2020;159:1935–48.

39. Brown RCH, Kelly D, Wilkinson D, et al. The scientific and ethical feasibility of immunity passports. Lancet Infect Dis 2020;21(3):e58–63.

40. US Department of Labor. Unemployment insurance weekly claims. 2020. Available at: https://www.dol.gov/sites/dolgov/files/OPA/newsreleases/ui-claims/20201122.pdf. Accessed March 6, 2021.

41. Nishihara R, Wu K, Lochhead P, et al. Long-term colorectal-cancer incidence and mortality after lower endoscopy. N Engl J Med 2013;369:1095–105.

42. Lee YC, Fann JC-Y, Chiang T-H, et al. Time to colonoscopy and risk of colorectal cancer in patients with positive results from fecal immunochemical tests. Clin Gastroenterol Hepatol 2019;17:1332–40.

43. Rutter CM, Kim JJ, Meester RGS, et al. Effect of time to diagnostic testing for breast, cervical, and colorectal cancer screening abnormalities on screening efficacy: a modeling study. Cancer Epidemiol Biomarkers Prev 2018;27:158–64.

44. Meester RG, Zauber AG, Doubeni CA, et al. Consequences of increasing time to colonoscopy examination after positive result from fecal colorectal cancer screening test. Clin Gastroenterol Hepatol 2016;14:1445–51.

45. Corley DA, Jensen CD, Quinn VP, et al. Association between time to colonoscopy after a positive fecal test result and risk of colorectal cancer and cancer stage at diagnosis. JAMA 2017;317:1631–41.

46. De Jonge L, Worthington J, Van Wifferen F, et al. Impact of the COVID-19 pandemic on faecal immunochemical test-based colorectal cancer screening programmes in Australia, Canada and the Netherlands: a comparative modelling study. Lancet Gastroenterol Hepatol 2021;6:304–14.

47. Morris EJA, Goldacre R, Spata E, et al. Impact of the COVID-19 pandemic on the detection and management of colorectal cancer in England: a population-based study. Lancet Gastroenterol Hepatol 2021;6(3):199–208.
48. Worthington J, Lew J-B, Feletto E, et al. Improving Australian National Bowel Cancer Screening Program outcomes through increased participation and cost-effective investment. PLoS One 2020;15:e0227899.
49. Keihanian T, Sharma P, Goyal J, et al. Telehealth utilization in gastroenterology clinics amid the COVID-19 pandemic: impact on clinical practice and gastroenterology training. Gastroenterology 2020;159:1598–601.
50. Dobrusin A, Hawa F, Gladshteyn M, et al. Gastroenterologists and patients report high satisfaction rates with telehealth services during the novel coronavirus 2019 pandemic. Clin Gastroenterol Hepatol 2020;18:2393–7.
51. Available at: https://realbusiness.co.uk/as-said-by-winston-churchill-never-waste-a-good-crisis/. Accessed March 7, 2021.
52. Morens DM, Fauci AS. Emerging pandemic diseases: how we got to COVID-19. Cell 2020;182:1077–92.

UNITED STATES POSTAL SERVICE®

Statement of Ownership, Management, and Circulation
(All Periodicals Publications Except Requester Publications)

1. Publication Title	2. Publication Number	3. Filing Date
GASTROINTESTINAL ENDOSCOPY CLINICS OF NORTH AMERICA	012 – 603	9/18/2021

4. Issue Frequency	5. Number of Issues Published Annually	6. Annual Subscription Price
JAN, APR, JUL, OCT	4	$363.00

7. Complete Mailing Address of Known Office of Publication (Not printer) (Street, city, county, state, and ZIP+4®)

ELSEVIER INC.
230 Park Avenue, Suite 800
New York, NY 10169

Contact Person
Malathi Samayan

Telephone (Include area code)
91-44-4299-4507

8. Complete Mailing Address of Headquarters or General Business Office of Publisher (Not printer)

ELSEVIER INC.
230 Park Avenue, Suite 800
New York, NY 10169

9. Full Names and Complete Mailing Addresses of Publisher, Editor, and Managing Editor (Do not leave blank)

Publisher (Name and complete mailing address)

DOLORES MELONI, ELSEVIER INC.
1600 JOHN F KENNEDY BLVD. SUITE 1800
PHILADELPHIA, PA 19103-2899

Editor (Name and complete mailing address)

KERRY HOLLAND, ELSEVIER INC.
1600 JOHN F KENNEDY BLVD. SUITE 1800
PHILADELPHIA, PA 19103-2899

Managing Editor (Name and complete mailing address)

PATRICK MANLEY, ELSEVIER INC.
1600 JOHN F KENNEDY BLVD. SUITE 1800
PHILADELPHIA, PA 19103-2899

10. Owner (Do not leave blank. If the publication is owned by a corporation, give the name and address of the corporation immediately followed by the names and addresses of all stockholders owning or holding 1 percent or more of the total amount of stock. If not owned by a corporation, give the names and addresses of the individual owners. If owned by a partnership or other unincorporated firm, give its name and address as well as those of each individual owner. If the publication is published by a nonprofit organization, give its name and address.)

Full Name	Complete Mailing Address
WHOLLY OWNED SUBSIDIARY OF REED/ELSEVIER, US HOLDINGS	1600 JOHN F KENNEDY BLVD. SUITE 1800 PHILADELPHIA, PA 19103-2899

11. Known Bondholders, Mortgagees, and Other Security Holders Owning or Holding 1 Percent or More of Total Amount of Bonds, Mortgages, or Other Securities. If none, check box ▶ ☐ None

Full Name	Complete Mailing Address
N/A	

12. Tax Status (For completion by nonprofit organizations authorized to mail at nonprofit rates) (Check one)
The purpose, function, and nonprofit status of this organization and the exempt status for federal income tax purposes:
☒ Has Not Changed During Preceding 12 Months
☐ Has Changed During Preceding 12 Months (Publisher must submit explanation of change with this statement)

PS Form 3526, July 2014 [Page 1 of 4 (see instructions page 4)] PSN 7530-01-000-9931 PRIVACY NOTICE: See our privacy policy on www.usps.com.

13. Publication Title		14. Issue Date for Circulation Data Below
GASTROINTESTINAL ENDOSCOPY CLINICS OF NORTH AMERICA		JULY 2021

15. Extent and Nature of Circulation		Average No. Copies Each Issue During Preceding 12 Months	No. Copies of Single Issue Published Nearest to Filing Date
a. Total Number of Copies (Net press run)		138	121
b. Paid Circulation (By Mail and Outside the Mail)	(1) Mailed Outside-County Paid Subscriptions Stated on PS Form 3541 (Include paid distribution above nominal rate, advertiser's proof copies, and exchange copies)	57	47
	(2) Mailed In-County Paid Subscriptions Stated on PS Form 3541 (Include paid distribution above nominal rate, advertiser's proof copies, and exchange copies)	0	0
	(3) Paid Distribution Outside the Mails Including Sales Through Dealers and Carriers, Street Vendors, Counter Sales, and Other Paid Distribution Outside USPS®	25	25
	(4) Paid Distribution by Other Classes of Mail Through the USPS (e.g., First-Class Mail®)	0	0
c. Total Paid Distribution (Sum of 15b (1), (2), (3), and (4))	▶	82	72
d. Free or Nominal Rate Distribution (By Mail and Outside the Mail)	(1) Free or Nominal Rate Outside-County Copies Included on PS Form 3541	40	32
	(2) Free or Nominal Rate In-County Copies Included on PS Form 3541	0	0
	(3) Free or Nominal Rate Copies Mailed at Other Classes Through the USPS (e.g., First-Class Mail)	0	0
	(4) Free or Nominal Rate Distribution Outside the Mail (Carriers or other means)	0	0
e. Total Free or Nominal Rate Distribution (Sum of 15d (1), (2), (3) and (4))	▶	40	32
f. Total Distribution (Sum of 15c and 15e)	▶	122	104
g. Copies not Distributed (See Instructions to Publishers #4 (page #3))	▶	16	17
h. Total (Sum of 15f and g)	▶	138	121
i. Percent Paid (15c divided by 15f times 100)	▶	67.21%	69.23%

* If you are claiming electronic copies, go to line 16 on page 3. If you are not claiming electronic copies, skip to line 17 on page 3.

16. Electronic Copy Circulation		Average No. Copies Each Issue During Preceding 12 Months	No. Copies of Single Issue Published Nearest to Filing Date
a. Paid Electronic Copies	▶		
b. Total Paid Print Copies (Line 15c) + Paid Electronic Copies (Line 16a)	▶		
c. Total Print Distribution (Line 15f) + Paid Electronic Copies (Line 16a)	▶		
d. Percent Paid (Both Print & Electronic Copies) (16b divided by 16c × 100)	▶		

☒ I certify that 50% of all my distributed copies (electronic and print) are paid above a nominal price.

17. Publication of Statement of Ownership
☒ If the publication is a general publication, publication of this statement is required. Will be printed in the OCTOBER 2021 issue of this publication.
☐ Publication not required.

18. Signature and Title of Editor, Publisher, Business Manager, or Owner

Malathi Samayan - Distribution Controller

Malathi Samayan

Date 9/18/2021

I certify that all information furnished on this form is true and complete. I understand that anyone who furnishes false or misleading information on this form or who omits material or information requested on the form may be subject to criminal sanctions (including fines and imprisonment) and/or civil sanctions (including civil penalties).

PS Form 3526, July 2014 (Page 3 of 4) PRIVACY NOTICE: See our privacy policy on www.usps.com.

Moving?

Make sure your subscription moves with you!

To notify us of your new address, find your **Clinics Account Number** (located on your mailing label above your name), and contact customer service at:

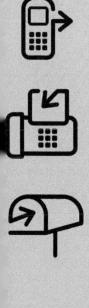

Email: journalscustomerservice-usa@elsevier.com

800-654-2452 (subscribers in the U.S. & Canada)
314-447-8871 (subscribers outside of the U.S. & Canada)

Fax number: 314-447-8029

Elsevier Health Sciences Division
Subscription Customer Service
3251 Riverport Lane
Maryland Heights, MO 63043

ELSEVIER

Printed and bound by CPI Group (UK) Ltd, Croydon, CR0 4YY

08/05/2025

01864700-0007